Special Educational Needs and Early Years Care and Education

For Baillière Tindall:

Publishing Manager: Inta Ozols
Project Development Manager: Karen Gilmour
Project Manager: Derek Robertson

Special Educational Needs in Early Years Care and Education

Lynda Littleboy CertEd RgNI
Early Years Consultant and Further and Adult
Education Teacher, West Sussex

Michael Reed MA(Ed) AdvDipEd CertEd
Educational Consultant, West Sussex

Jill Thompson NVQ (Training) AdvDip
Trainer, Assessor, Internal and External Verifier,
West Sussex

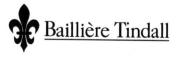

Baillière Tindall

EDINBURGH LONDON NEW YORK PHILADELPHIA ST LOUIS SYDNEY TORONTO 2000

BAILLIÈRE TINDALL
An imprint of Harcourt Publishers Limited

First published 2000

ISBN 07020 2385 X

British Library Cataloguing in Publication Data
A catalogue record for this book is available from the British
Library

Library of Congress Cataloging in Publication Data
A catalog record for this book is available from the Library
of Congress

The
publisher's
policy is to use
paper manufactured
from sustainable forests

Printed in China

CONTENTS

INTRODUCTION

This book is intended as a starting point to assist you in developing and refining your professional practice in the field of early years care and education.

The book is aimed at early years workers and students who require information about policy and practice, as well as an explanation of the impact that special needs may have on children, their families and the education they receive.

You may be involved in obtaining a recognised qualification in early years care and education. This may be at a college-based course or an NVQ qualification carried out in the workplace. You may be following a course of study designed by a voluntary sector organisation or you may be attending training which considers specific aspects of support for children with special educational needs. We have included tasks and exercises throughout the book which we hope will extend your knowledge and understanding, as well as provide evidence that may be used for an NVQ award.

Aims

The aims of the book are as follows:

- *To increase your knowledge and understanding of special educational needs in the early years*
- *To increase your knowledge and understanding of policy and practice within the workplace and to explore ways to 'include' young children with special educational needs*
- *To consider good practice and strategies that may be introduced to assist children and their families*
- *To gain an insight into the way in which children with special educational needs are supported in the workplace.*
- *To engage in tasks which are based on case studies of children with special educational needs.*

Key issues

The book addresses these issues:

- *The difference between a **condition**, a **physical disability** and a **special need***

- *How a particular condition like asthma, an injury like a broken leg or a long stay in hospital can affect a child's learning and educational progress*
- *Parents' rights in relation to their children with special educational needs*
- *The difference between **identification** and **assessment** of special educational needs*
- *Procedures to assess and provide for young children with special educational needs*
- *Types of special schools and special provision*
- *Different professionals who help children with special educational needs*
- *How children with different conditions have experienced different forms of support.*

An experience of learning

We all learn in different ways. Our learning is the result of a range of experiences, which influence the way we think and react in different situations. Our culture, our religion and where we live all play a part in the way we experience learning.

Parents make a difference to the way we learn. They provide more than food, love, care and warmth. They provide the boundaries that help us to understand right and wrong. They provide a model for the way we act towards others and they are our first point of contact with the adult world.

As we grow, we form a picture of the world around us. We learn what is expected of us in terms of social norms. We learn that not everyone is the same. Some people are friendly, others cold, some are athletic, others find physical activity more difficult. Some have particular talents like a marvellous singing voice or the ability to paint or draw. Some have individual talents such as caring for others or a personality that keeps them smiling though all forms of adversity. We are starting to accept this diversity and value individuals for what they *can* do, rather than condemn them for what they are unable to do.

Special educational needs (SEN) is a term that is most often used to describe an individual who requires support in order to maximise his or her learning. The terms 'handicapped', 'dull', 'stupid', 'sub-normal' and 'thick' are no longer appropriate as we start to consider ways that children may be *included* in learning activities, rather than excluded because they are different and or have special requirements. We are not suggesting that everyone is the same, just that we should celebrate diversity.

It can be argued that attitudes towards children with special needs have changed over the years. People are more tolerant and have a greater understanding about particular conditions. Such change has taken time and has been influenced by many factors.

Some changes have been driven by the government which has altered the law to enforce particular practices. The last Disability Discrimination Act is a case in point. Some changes have been influenced by society modifying its attitude as a result of publicity or public feeling. Some changes are the result of parents taking action themselves and some are the result of developments in educational practice. Some have been influenced by the media which informs parents of their rights and plays an active role in highlighting the needs of children, even raising funds to assist particular groups in society.

So, there are a variety of things that have promoted change in attitude and practice. When you read the first two chapters which deal with the historical factors that have influenced the way we respond to children today, remember that change is a *process* and not just a series of events. Attitudes *do* matter therefore the way *we* respond to children with special educational needs will contribute to the change process.

Terminology

Note that child care and education can take place in many different *settings*: at nursery, at playgroup, in a reception class at school, in day care centres, and in a childminder's home or in a child's home with a nanny. All these settings are child care *providers*. Many different people may be involved in child care and education: teachers, nannies, key workers, classroom assistants and childminders. As a group these are often referred to as *early years workers*.

ACKNOWLEDGEMENTS

The authors would like to acknowledge the help and support given to them by friends, colleagues and children and to those friends and colleagues who gave their time to read first drafts and to comment upon the book. Thanks also go to the parents and children who allowed them to gain an insight into the way that they were supported in order to meet the children's special educational needs.

1: WHAT ARE SPECIAL EDUCATIONAL NEEDS?

Key Points & Introduction

- A current definition of special educational needs
- Physical and learning disabilities
- The difference between disability and handicap
- The importance of our attitude towards children with special educational needs.

It is important to consider a current definition of special needs (the historical developments which have led to our current understanding of the term are discussed in Chapter 2). A Government Green Paper called *Excellence in Schools*, published in 1998, provides a useful starting point. It says:

> 'The term "special educational needs" can be misleading and lead to unhelpful assumptions. It may suggest that children with SEN are a readily defined group, with common characteristics. It is sometimes used as though it applied only to the 3% of pupils with a statement of SEN. It is sometimes used of children from disadvantaged families. All this is far from the truth.'

It goes on to offer a definition:

> 'The law says that a child has special educational needs if he or she has: a learning difficulty (i.e. a significantly greater difficulty in learning than the majority of children of the same age, or a disability which makes it difficult to use the educational facilities generally provided locally); and if that learning difficulty calls for special educational provision (i.e. provision additional to, or different from, that made generally for children of the same age in local schools).
>   Whether or not a child has SEN will therefore depend both on the individual and on local circumstances. It may be entirely consistent with the law for a child to be said to have special educational needs in one school, but not in another.'

Some definitions

There is no such group as 'The Disabled'! There are, however, young children who have different conditions and differing needs. Be less concerned about using the correct terms and be more concerned with the attitudes and actions behind your words. Think about ways you can include children rather than concentrating on conditions which may exclude them.

Some conditions result in a *physical disability*. Physical disabilities relate to the body and the senses. Hearing and sight impairment are physical disabilities. As we get older, we all become subject to a variety of physical disabilities!

Other conditions may result in a *learning disability*. These disabilities relate to the way we receive information and communicate with others. It is also about the pace of how we learn about things around us.

Physical and learning disabilities are not necessarily permanent. People change and make progress. There may be factors, such as family crisis or bereavement, which create a temporary problem. Many children may have a learning difficulty at some time in their early education and schooling.

Bear in mind that conditions are not always visible. Emotional damage is not easily seen and low self-esteem can be hard to identify. Epilepsy and deafness are two examples of physical conditions which are not immediately obvious. All these factors can cause a child to need additional help with learning.

What about the term 'handicap'?

A *handicap* is the result of having a condition in a society which is not suitably adapted. Not having a ramp to provide physical access for a person in a wheelchair is a handicap. The person himself does not have a handicap. When you visit a country and are unable to speak the language you are handicapped.

Attitudes

We all have to be aware of the fact that our behaviour towards children with special needs conveys a message to all the children in our care. You might inadvertently be giving the impression that disability is something to be cured. You might be giving the impression that people with special needs should be cared for and we should always provide for them, rather than promote their independence. Hopefully you will give the view that disabled people are independent, capable, take pride in their achievements and can control their own destiny.

It is important to portray people with special needs in a positive light when providing toys, creating displays and using illustrations in early years settings. Just as you might have a variety of coloured paints so that children can portray different skin tones, you can provide dolls, toys and other playthings which have positive representations of people with a disability.

Conclusion

In 1997, a survey of schools indicated that 18% of pupils – 1.5 million children – had special educational needs. This statistic must make all early years practitioners consider the importance of recognising and providing for children with special needs. Your role in the early identification of potential special needs may be vital to children's later development.

2: UNDERSTANDING THE FRAMEWORK FOR SPECIAL EDUCATIONAL PROVISION

Key Points & Introduction

- The Education Act 1944
- The Warnock Committee and Report (Department of Education and Science 1978)
- The Education Act 1981

- The Children Act 1989
- The National Curriculum
- The Code of Practice 1994
- Nursery vouchers 1996
- The Green Paper 1998.

Workplace practice in relation to children with special educational needs has changed over time. In addition, attitudes towards handicap and disability have also changed. There has been a movement away from the concept of disease as a cause of disability towards a view in which the educational and social needs of the child are paramount, irrespective of the condition which creates the needs. Today, there is an emphasis on providing whatever the child needs to be included within educational and social activities. These developments have occurred largely within the second half of the twentieth century.

Changing attitudes

The Education Act 1944

To consider how attitudes and practice have changed we will start with the 1944 Education Act. The Act provided a significant and radical approach to the education of children, stating that children with special needs should have the opportunity to be educated alongside their peers and that the views of parents should be recognised. However, in practice it was medical services rather than educationalists, or indeed parents, who took the lead in determining what provision should be made available to children. There was a clear emphasis on fitting children with special needs into different 'categories of handicap'. In the Act these catagories ranged from 'blind' to 'deaf' and 'delicate'. Even epilepsy was seen as a specific category of handicap. For those children who were considered to have profound learning difficulties the term *uneducable* was used and they were *diagnosed* rather than *assessed*. Parents played little part in the process of identification and assessment of their children's needs. They were given little support and few choices about their children's education.

Special schools

By the 1970s a different form of categorisation was being used. This related to the types of educational provision that were available. Children with special needs were considered 'educationally sub-normal' and would usually attend a special school. Children were classed as either *educationally sub-normal (mild)* or *educationally subnormal (severe)* and then sent to the corresponding type of school. It was not until the early 1970s that the term 'uneducable' was at last removed from official records. This proved to be a turning point in the move from a medical diagnosis to an educational assessment and a staged process of intervention.

The Warnock Committee and Report

During the mid 1970s a government Committee chaired by Mary Warnock, now Dame Mary Warnock, was established. It was charged with the task of reviewing the whole process of identification, intervention and support for people with special educational needs. When the committee reported its findings there was significant interest in their recommendations, particularly in how special needs should be identified and in how provision should be made for children.

Other countries, such as the USA, were also making changes at this time. This included giving rights to parents and suggesting that educationalists should design individual educational plans that would give a detailed account of how a child with special needs would be taught. When the Warnock Report was finally published it recommended a formal staged process that should be followed to identify and assess a child's special educational needs. This process would not be led by medical agencies, but by groups of professionals working together in partnership with parents. The report also recommended that children should have the protection of a *statement* (a formal record) of their needs.

It could be argued that the Warnock Committee and the resulting report played a significant part in influencing change. It certainly acted as a starting point for the development of interagency working. However, it could also be argued that the report retained too many of the established practices, which gave significant decision-making powers to professionals and few rights or representation to parents.

The Education Act 1981

A number of key points from the Warnock Report were contained within the 1981 Education Act, which came into force in 1983. This provided a structure for multi-disciplinary assessment and provided parents with the opportunity to play a part in deciding the educational provision most suitable for their child. The Act placed a duty upon Local Education Authorities (LEAs) to consider the educational requirements of children with special needs and provided the right of appeal for parents who were concerned about the provision offered to their child. It gave schools the opportunity to review their early intervention policy and practice. It recognised the need, not only for identification, but also for intervention by health, social services and education departments working together.

Criticisms of the 1981 Act

1. Although parents were given rights and opportunities to take part in assessment this was limited to participation rather than decision-making.
2. There were disputes between professionals and LEAs, usually over resources or provision. Many disputes reached the stage of a formal appeal to a local committee and thereafter to the Secretary of State for Education. In a number of cases this resulted in decisions being made by the Courts. On a more positive note, the educational aims of the 1981 Act were enforced by legal precedent.
3. The Act was not accompanied by additional finance to LEAs in order to implement its recommendations. The result was that LEAs around the country provided very different resources. Some did their utmost to work in partnership with parents and to look carefully at each child's individual needs. Others provided only a limited response to the 1981 Act.

This state of affairs continued throughout the 1980s and the procedures were subject to a number of reviews by Her Majesty's Inspectorate and a Government Select Committee. The reviews concluded that the system was cumbersome and that, although there was an emphasis upon *inclusive education* and integrating children with special needs into mainstream schools, there was little real progress towards effective choice for parents and children. In addition, during the period between 1983 and 1996 there was a steady increase in the number of children identified as having special educational needs and provided with a statement.

The Children Act 1989

Even the advent of the Children Act 1989, which came into force in 1991, did little to integrate the principles and practice of the 1981 Education Act. The notion of interdisciplinary assessment and meeting needs was present, though once again the legal definition emphasised a negative model of disability. In the Children Act, a child is said to be disabled if

> 'he is blind, deaf or dumb or suffers from mental disorder of any kind or is substantially and permanently handicapped by illness, injury or congenital deformity or such other disability as may be prescribed.'

However, it could be argued that all of these developments were at least providing a focus for change. Parents of children with special needs were starting to lobby educationalists and demanding that their voice was heard by those in government. The media was providing high profile coverage of the issues. Many European countries and the USA were developing legislation that gave rights and full representation to parents. Schools were also becoming skilled in supporting pupils with special needs.

Early identification was recognised as important and a number of projects aimed at young children and their parents were established. One example was the *Portage home visiting service* which realised one of the aims of the Warnock Committee in promoting the notion of parents and professionals working together. There was an increasing emphasis upon integrating children in mainstream schools and parents' input into the assessment process was recognised.

The National Curriculum

With the advent of the National Curriculum, special educational needs were thrown into sharp profile. The National Curriculum was hailed as a programme for all and there was a clear attempt to include *all* children, unless there were quite specific educational reasons for exclusion. Ongoing assessment was seen as an essential part of the new curriculum with children assessed at different stages of their educational career. Alongside these initiatives the government introduced many changes in the way schools were managed and financed and regular school inspection by the Office for Standards in Education (OfSTED) began.

The Code of Practice on the Identification and Assessment of Special Educational Needs 1994

With such considerable reform of the whole educational service in England and

Wales, it was a natural progression to introduce measures for a national approach to special needs. Therefore in 1994, the government introduced the Code of Practice on children with special educational needs. Under the Code educationalists were required to identify children with special needs, assess the extent of their difficulties and seek outside professional advice in order to minimise such difficulties. They were required to put in place procedures for formal assessment of pupils and to participate in the design of a formal record or statement of special educational needs. Throughout the process there was a particular emphasis on the way that parents were informed and involved.

Nursery vouchers

The introduction of the nursery voucher scheme in 1996 gave the Code increased relevance in early years settings. Early years providers receiving government funding through the scheme were required to follow the Code of Practice. With a change of government in 1997, the emphasis on special educational needs in the early years has continued. Although the voucher scheme was disbanded, it was replaced by a requirement for Local Authorities to prepare *Early Years Development Plans*. These plans outline the way different providers of early years education should work together. Importantly in relation to children with special needs, these plans address how Local Authorities can support early identification and provision for young children with special educational needs.

Looking to the future

A further development occurred at the start of 1998. This was a government Green Paper intended as a framework for consultation on how to improve provision for children with special needs, looking forward into the new millennium. The Green Paper tackles many of the issues raised in this chapter and presents a realistic way forward in order to support children with special educational needs.

The Green Paper places significant emphasis on raising the standards that children achieve in schools. It argues that good provision for SEN does not mean a sympathetic acceptance of low achievement. It means a tough-minded determination to show that children with SEN are capable of excellence. It argues that, when schools respond to children in this way, teachers are more likely to set high standards for all pupils.

The Green Paper suggests that the great majority of children with SEN will, as adults, contribute economically and socially as members of society. Schools have to prepare all children for their future roles. This is a sound reason for educating children with SEN, as far as possible, with their peers. Where all children are included as equal partners in the school community, the benefits are felt by all.

The Green Paper sets out an approach for improving the achievement of children with special educational needs in the early years:

> 'All our programmes for raising standards will reflect this, starting from pre-school provision, building on the information provided by the new arrangements for baseline assessment when children start in primary school, and leading to improved ways of tackling problems with early literacy and numeracy;'

Parental contributions are also given high priority within the Green Paper:

> 'For many parents, learning of their child's problems will be a devastating blow. Nothing can entirely remove the pressures they will face, but much can be done to share them. There is no reason why any parent should feel the sense of not knowing where to turn which has been the experience of too many. In all our actions bearing on special educational needs, we shall take account of the effects on parents and families. We recognise that some parents will need support from a range of statutory and voluntary agencies if they are to help their children to flourish.'

Importantly, the Green Paper sets specific goals to which the government will aspire, and within this framework there are specific references to the early years.

> 'The policies set out in *Excellence in Schools* for raising standards, particularly in the early years, will be beginning to reduce the number of children who need long-term special educational provision.
>
> There will be stronger and more consistent arrangements in place across the country for the early identification of SEN.
>
> The best way to tackle educational disadvantage is to get in early. When educational failure becomes entrenched, pupils can move from demoralisation to disruptive behaviour and truancy. But early diagnosis and appropriate intervention improve the prospects of children with special educational needs, and reduce the need for expensive intervention later on. For some children, giving more effective attention to early signs of difficulties can prevent the development of SEN.
>
> The majority of children with the most severe disabilities will be identified well before they start school; but health and social services professionals should also look for other factors which may lead to educational disadvantage. District Health Authorities and NHS Trusts are under a duty to bring to the LEA's

attention any child under five who they think has SEN. An integrated approach by child health professionals, social services and education staff is needed right from the start, making full use of the children's services planning process.

To widen the options available, we want to encourage innovative partnerships between statutory and voluntary agencies. Multi-agency support for children with SEN will be a priority in our new pilot programme for early excellence centres.

From September 1998, all children will be assessed as they begin their primary education. Baseline assessment will not on its own establish whether individual pupils have special educational needs. But it will be crucial in helping to show where a child has problems which need attention – whether these arise from special needs, or from family or emotional difficulties. It should show teachers those pupils who need a targeted teaching strategy or further classroom based assessment, perhaps leading to specific support from the school or from other agencies.'

Conclusion

For those involved in the early years, the Green Paper provides a degree of optimism in relation to early identification and appropriate provision. It addresses many of the issues raised in this chapter and sets the scene for the remainder of this book. We hope that, following consultation, many of the proposals outlined in the Green Paper will be implemented.

3: THE CODE OF PRACTICE

- Duties of providers under the Code of Practice
- Principles underpinning the Code
- Practices and procedures

- Special needs policies
- The five stages leading to a statement of special educational needs
- Named persons.

The full title of the Code of Practice is 'The Code of Practice on the Identification and Assessment of Special Educational Needs'. It came into force on 1st September 1994 and was intended to address the needs of some 20% of children who, at some time in their education, require special educational provision. With regard to young children the Code states:

'Children under five will be assessed utilising information from similar sources [to those used for older children] and settings that provide for young children have a duty to comply with the Code to ensure that children receive the best possible provision to meet their needs. Early years settings will be expected to follow broadly the same procedures for identifying and meeting special education needs as those providing for children of compulsory school age. The involvement of health professionals will be particularly crucial for younger children where data as to the child's "educational" stage is not yet available.'

Statements in the early years

It is rare for children under 2 years to receive a formal statement of educational needs, but where the decision is made to issue a statement this will usually be because of the child's complex needs or to provide access to specific services (e.g. Portage). To comply with the Code of Practice information should be collected by early years workers. Information needed to issue a statement includes:

- *Anything available about the child with a clear specification of the child's special educational needs*
- *A record of the views of the parents and those of any relevant professionals*
- *A clear account of the services being offered, including the contribution of the education services and details of any educational objectives that have been set, the contributions of any statutory and voluntary agencies and a description of the arrangements for monitoring and review.*

Duties under the Code of Practice

The Code of Practice sets out the principles which underpin the duties of educational providers to children with special educational needs:

- 'the needs of all pupils who may have special education needs either throughout or at any time during their school careers must be addressed; the Code recognizes that there is a continuum of needs and a continuum of provision, which may be made in a wide variety of different forms
- children with special educational needs require the greatest possible access to a broad and balanced education, including the National Curriculum
- the needs of most pupils will be met in the mainstream, and without a statutory assessment or statement of special educational needs. Children with special educational needs, including children with statements of special educational needs, should, where appropriate and taking into account the wishes of their parents, be educated alongside their peers in mainstream schools
- even before he or she reaches compulsory school age a child may have special education needs requiring the intervention of the LEA as well as the health services
- the knowledge, views and experience of parents are vital. Effective assessment and provision will be secured where there is the greatest possible degree of partnership between parents and their children and schools, LEAs and other agencies.'

The Code also describes the practices and procedures essential in pursuit of these principles:

- 'all children with special educational needs should be identified and assessed as early as possible and as quickly as is consistent with thoroughness
- provision for all children with special educational needs should be made by the most appropriate agency. In most cases this will be the child's mainstream school, working in partnership with the child's parents: no statutory assessment will be necessary
- where needed LEAs must make assessment and statements in accordance with the prescribed time limits; must write clear and thorough statements, setting out the child's educational and non-educational needs, the objectives to be secured, the provision to be made and the arrangements for monitoring and review, and ensure the annual review of the special educational provision arranged for the child and the updating and monitoring of educational targets.

- special educational provision will be most effective when those responsible take into account the ascertainable wishes of the child concerned, considered in the light of his or her age and understanding
- there must be close cooperation between all the agencies concerned and a multi-disciplinary approach to the resolution of issues.'

In addition, the Code requires all settings to have a *policy statement* which sets out how staff ensure they are providing for all children, and how they offer support for families during the statementing process.

Putting the code into practice

Special needs policies

All early years workers can play a part in helping to identify and provide for children with special educational needs. All staff in every setting providing care and education for children need to be aware of the Code and how it affects their provision. To guarantee a unified approach throughout the setting, providers should design a policy to which all staff are happy to subscribe and supply any supporting information or resources to assist staff and parents. The policy should consider:

- *How concerns about children with potential special needs will be identified*
- *How such concerns will be related to the parents and how action will be taken following discussions with the parents*
- *Who will coordinate an initial plan for monitoring and assessing a particular child, and how to include any other professionals at this stage*
- *Who will decide upon review dates and who will keep parents informed*
- *Who will construct and agree with the parents a detailed plan and timetable for the assessment process*
- *Who will ensure the Code of Practice is being adhered to*
- *Who will coordinate a review of policy, both generally and in relation to individual children*
- *Who will collate information about specific conditions, syndromes and illnesses*
- *Who will coordinate training, either specific or general.*

Recent guidelines suggest that all providers should inform parents of the provision made for children with special educational needs as part of the written information which is sent out when children start at the setting.

A five stage approach

The Code of Practice uses five stages to identify and provide for children with special educational needs. At each stage the following should occur:

- Information is gathered from as full a range of sources as possible to identify the child's strengths and weaknesses, taking account of views of the parents and the child as appropriate
- Individual plans are then made using the information to set targets and to agree dates and methods for review
- At each review it is decided whether the child should continue to receive similar support, whether support is no longer required or that the next stage is triggered and the child receives a different level or type of support.

Named Persons

As we have discussed, the Code takes account of parental views. It also makes provision for parental support mechanisms. One such mechanism is the Named Person system. A Named Person can be anyone nominated by the family to help them deal with the complex procedures and many professionals involved with their child with special educational needs. A Named Person can be anyone known to the family – a teacher or other professional who knows the child and is willing to assist in supporting the family. A Named Person may be asked to attend meetings with parents and teachers, head teachers and other professionals.

LEAs in many areas of the UK have introduced a programme whereby volunteers become Named Persons and are trained to help families. This training will include familiarisation with the local procedures, information about different schools and specialist schools, listening skills and guidelines to help them in their role. It is important to highlight that a Named Person's purpose is not to give advice or make decisions, but to act as a sounding board, identifying the options and encouraging families to think about the various choices. Volunteers' details may be held by the LEA who are able to assign a Named Person on request by a family.

Both the Code itself and the *Parents Guide to the Code* are available in a variety of languages, in Braille and on audio cassette. These can be obtained free from the DFEE.

Conclusion

The Code of Practice was introduced to create a unified approach to providing for children with special educational needs. Prior to this, the support that children and parents received very much depended on where they lived and their Local Authority's policies.

The Code sets out the duties of providers to the children in their care and also makes clear a number of procedures which should be followed when assessing the needs of children. In particular, the Code uses a five stage approach leading to the production of a formal statement of special educational needs for a particular child and it also requires that all settings create their own special needs policy. The Code makes a point of involving parents and provides a Named Person System to help parents through the complexities that they encounter.

The Way Forward

Early years

There have recently been further developments within the field of special education and the inclusion of pupils with special educational needs. In terms of the early years, the most recent change is that the Desirable Learning Outcomes are to be replaced by Early Learning Goals. This is the result of an extensive process of consultation with all manner of practitioners and interested parties. The result was published by QCA and the DfEE in October 1999. The goals set out to assist practitioners in arriving at what children should learn in their early years of education at nursery or school. The principle of support for children with special educational needs remains and there is an emphasis on removing barriers to learning and preventing learning difficulties from developing. A copy of the document may be obtained from the Qualifications and Curriculum Authority (Tel.: 01787 884444) or can be downloaded from the QCA web site at www. qca.org.uk/.

Inclusive trends

As many as 80% of children with a condition such as Down's syndrome or hearing impairment are educated in mainstream schools. The identification of children with special needs is becoming more focused upon those in the early stages of their school career. It is suggested that just over 53% of children who have recently been issued with a Statement of Special Educational Needs are between five and ten years of age. The volume of Statements has increased between 1993 (2.3%) and 1999 (3.1%). The trend is towards including such 'statemented' pupils in mainstream schools.

A recent professorship for inclusion has been established at the Cambridge Institute of Education. The Institute intends to produce an 'index for inclusive schools'. The index will explore how a school can create an inclusive culture amongst staff and pupils, design and develop inclusive policies and promote inclusive practice.

The government have announced that they intend to place significant sums of money into the development of literacy support, inclusive education for children with emotional and behavioural difficulties and the professional development of teachers.

Legislation

The Code of Practice is to be reviewed. It is thought that this will be finalised by 2001. Consultation has begun and it is suggested that the volume of Statements should be reduced by 2% with the introduction of the revised code.

Finally . . .

It is gratifying to report that there have been recent positive changes within the field of inlcusive education. We hope this demonstrates that meeting special educational needs is not something static and resistant to change. Indeed, we would argue that changing attitudes to practice is important if we are to strive to assist those with special educational needs. In 1978 the Warnock Committee suggested that assessment was a process rather than an event. We think that meeting special educational needs is a process and not a single event. It involves changes in attitude, funding, professional expertise and a commitment to inclusive education in the early years and beyond.

4: DOCUMENTS RELATING TO PRACTICE

Key Points & Introduction

- The Welcome Booklet
- The Parent/Carer and Provider's Contract
- Suggestions for behaviour management policies
- Evaluating a document.

An early years setting will require a variety of clear and concise documents for use by both staff and parents. We have already considered the special needs policy which settings must create to fulfil the requirements of the Code of Practice. Other documents which a setting may consider necessary are a Welcome Booklet to be given to the parents of new children, a contract between the setting and the child's parents or carer outlining the responsibilities that the parties have to each other and a behaviour management policy. All these should be working documents and everyone involved with the setting should be aware of their contents, willing and able to adapt their practice accordingly.

The Welcome Booklet

The type of provision offered by different settings will vary in as many ways as those settings themselves vary: because of staff expertise, the children, funding, premises, resources and equipment, for example.

The Welcome Booklet is like a prospectus. It provides an opportunity for the setting to 'sell' its provision to parents. It may be a particularly important source of information for parents of children with special educational needs. These parents will be looking for a group that concentrates on inclusive provision. They will want to see that the group provides opportunities for children to enjoy themselves whilst learning, experiencing and developing to their own potential. This is good practice for all children, not just children with special needs. For instance, a parent assessing the provision for their child could read about the use of an interest table with adults and children talking about the objects and using all their senses to explore the objects. A child with special needs can be included in this activity without anything 'special' being done for them.

Contents of the Welcome Booklet

The Welcome Booklet could contain all or some of the information set out below:

- *The setting's identifying mark* – a logo, picture or something else which represents the setting's name.
- *The aims of the setting* – for example: 'The aim of the group is to offer a safe, caring and well-resourced environment, with trained, committed staff, enabling young children to learn and grow through play and experience governed by an early years curriculum designed to encourage them to reach their individual full potential.'
- *A brief history of the group* – when it was set up, who by, any special landmark occasions or anniversaries.
- *Practical information* – opening times, contact names, addresses, telephone numbers, fees (when and how payable), types of refreshment provided, safety rules and requirements, for example, soft shoes, children not allowed in a particular area.
- *Registration form* – sheet requesting information, including medical details, parent's contact numbers, information about the child's likes, dislikes, fears, favourite toys, stories, activities, family and extended family members, pets, friends who already attend the group and a space for parents to comment on anything else they feel is appropriate.
- *Special needs policy* – details of how the group welcomes children with special needs and will provide an integrated curriculum for them. A brief description of the Code of Practice and a promise to abide by it may be helpful.
- *Settling-in policy* – how parents are encouraged to integrate their children, the number and timing of pre-attendance visits, a suggestion of how long parents might like to stay with their child to ensure they are settled in, details of any key worker system, when and how parents will be informed about how the child has settled.
- *The curriculum on offer* – the sorts of activities with a brief description of how these link to educational outcomes, examples of projects, outings, visitors to the group for example.
- *The basic routine* – what happens when and why.
- *The staff* – this could include brief biographies and photographs.
- *Illustrations* – photographs, pictures produced by the children, computer graphics.
- *Anecdotes* – short quotes from children and parents about their time at the group.

- *Date of production and any updates* – to ensure current information is available.

The parent/carer and provider's contract

A contract which sets out the parent or carer's and provider's responsibilities can be a useful document. It should be clear, comprehensive and easy to understand. It should contain or make reference to the policy documents relating to the setting. When parents sign the contract they should be made aware that they are accepting the terms of these policies.

Accessibility

The contract must be equally accessible to *all* parents. This may mean:

- *Providing copies on tape, in another language or in Braille*
- *Having staff available to go through the contract with parents, explaining clearly to ensure their understanding.*

Sample contracts

Two sample contracts are given below. Do not copy these documents. It is important to adapt them to your own needs.

Sample 1

The setting will provide:

1 *For children's physical needs*
- *A safe, clean, hygienic, warm, caring, friendly environment*
- *Accessible and appropriate toilet facilities*
- *A safe and stimulating outside play area*
- *Evidence of a first aid certificate*

- *Safe transport arrangements (seatbelts, appropriate insurance)*
- *A ratio of one member of staff to two children for outings*
- *Obtain permission from parents prior to outings*
- *Staff that have been police checked*
- *Food and drinks*
- *Provision for sleep or rest as appropriate.*

2 *Staff that*
- *Have relevant training and experience*
- *Are able to recognise and fulfil children's needs*
- *Have been police checked and registered with Social Services.*

3 *A curriculum that*
- *Ensures children are able to learn through experience and play*
- *Includes display of children's work*
- *Provides stimulating toys and resources for girls and boys*
- *Uses a variety of craft materials to suit all ages and stages*
- *Includes observation, record keeping and reporting to parents as appropriate*
- *Provides protective clothes for messy activities.*

4 *Policies that cover*
- *Behaviour management*
- *Settling in procedures*
- *Equal opportunities*
- *Special needs*
- *Staff employment and management*
- *Complaints*
- *Fire*
- *Child protection*
- *Confidentiality*
- *Rules and regulations*
- *Health, safety and emergency procedures*
- *Cooperation with other providers (toddler groups, nursery, schools).*

Parents agree to:

- *Give notice of holiday dates as soon as possible but at least two weeks beforehand*

- Give half a term's notice if removing the child from the provider – a full half-term's fees will be due if notice is not given
- Keep the child away if they have any infectious diseases and advise the provider accordingly
- Provide information regarding food likes and dislikes, including any allergies
- Advise the provider of any changes to the child's routine when being collected by another person or at a different time
- Provide full information regarding the child's medical history, including any allergies, details of the GP or health visitor, details of any medication the child is to receive together with permission and information about how this should be administered
- Provide full registration details including emergency contacts, a record of which will be revised and kept up to date as necessary
- Receive notice of and give evidence of permission for outings as appropriate
- Make payments promptly, weekly in arrears
- Make additional payments for late collections, and such other arrangements as may be agreed between the provider and parents (payment will be by cheque, cash, direct debit or as agreed)
- Take a view on and input into planning activities which will form the curriculum being implemented with the child and which will work towards the learning outcomes recognised by the DFEE
- Receive information about and take part in discussions relating to unacceptable behaviour, including how such behaviour will be managed – physical punishment will never be used
- Provide full information regarding any special needs the child has and take part in discussions about how to support such needs
- Approach the provider at any time with problems or concerns
- Be advised of Social Services' checks and health and safety inspections and their outcome
- Accept responsibility for damage to any of the child's clothing or belongings brought to the setting
- Be contacted as soon as possible in the event of any emergency and to be advised of the whereabouts of the child
- Abide by policies relating to fire, health and safety, behaviour, child protection, complaints, settling in, equal opportunities, confidentiality.

Parents will have a right of access to any information kept on their child or family and will be allowed to spend time with their child as agreed with the setting

Sample 2

Providers and parents agree to their commitment as set out below:

- Providers will deliver, to the best of their ability, a safe, happy, warm and caring environment where each child is treated as an individual and is encouraged to reach their full potential through a curriculum designed to meet the DFEE's learning outcomes. There will be suitable equipment for all ages and stages of child development. All staff will have access to training and in-service training. A variety of meals, drinks and snacks will be provided to suit each child's needs. Children will have access to any comfort objects that they require.
- Details of the curriculum operated by the group will be published regularly and parents will be encouraged to discuss and comment on this. A prospectus will be published.
- Providers will deliver a service between the hours of 9 am to 12 noon, Monday to Friday, term time only, excluding Bank Holidays.
- There is an expectation that all children will participate in every activity and will come clothed accordingly.
- The setting will operate under Social Services' guidelines and regulations, offering a staff to child ratio of 1:8 as laid down by The Children Act 1989.
- The provider requires written notice of half a term, or payment in lieu. Fees will be paid half-termly in advance and bills will be provided in advance. The setting will provide details of payments to be made, how and when such payments should be made. Parents agree to pay promptly. Payment is required for times when a child is away from the group due to sickness or holiday, unless prior arrangement is made with the group in specific circumstances.
- Parents will give notice of the child's absence for any reason including illness and the setting will not accept any child who has been unwell during the previous 24 hours. If there is any doubt about the child's fitness to attend the group the supervisor will make the final decision.
- The provider will care for children within the stated times. Parents will be responsible for their children before and after each session and are also responsible for collecting their children promptly, or for arranging for their child's collection. Any changes to the normal routine are to be

advised to the group and anyone unknown to the group may be asked for identification.

- The setting will operate the following policies and parents agree to abide by them: health and safety, behaviour, equal opportunities, special needs, admissions and settling in, parent involvement, confidentiality, staffing and student, emergency and evaluation, child protection, curriculum plans, complaints procedures. A copy of each policy operated by the setting is displayed within the building and these are also available to all parents upon request.

- The provider will offer parents opportunities to spend time settling their child and to participate in any activity or to offer any specialist skills which they feel may be of value to the group. The group encourages all parents to view any performances in which their children are involved, and also to support any fund raising or other activities. All funds raised are used directly to benefit the children. The group encourages parental involvement in the everyday running of the setting and acknowledges the right of parents to be involved with their children in whatever ways are agreed as suitable.

- The setting expects all parents to read and understand the group's child protection policy as the group are legally required to report any concerns to Social Services. The group operates a complaints procedure, a copy of which is available. However any complaints should initially be brought to the attention of the group's supervisor. Complaints will be dealt with within 7 days. If a dispute is not resolved within that time, the complaint will be passed to the local Social Services Department for resolution within an agreed time limit.

- The provision complies with The Children Act and Local Authority regulations.

- The setting will provide outings which are suitably supervised and notified to parents. Parental involvement is encouraged and parental consent will always be sought.

- The provider will keep records of all relevant medical details, contact numbers and needs of the child. Parents agree to supply this information as required.

- The setting will provide opportunities to meet with parents to discuss the progress of their children and to provide mutual support in the event of any problems or concerns.

- The provision and parents will cooperate fully at all times in the best interests of the children.

Behaviour management policies

All settings, but particularly those with SEN children will require a behaviour management policy. Problem behaviour may include unacceptable, unpredictable, and even unsafe behaviour. A well thought out policy will have the scope to deal with poor behaviour from any child. It is essential that all children see that unacceptable behaviour remains unacceptable whoever is the perpetrator. Behaviour can be made 'understandable', but not 'excusable', if exhibited by a child with special needs.

Behaviour is an area of particular concern to parents. A behaviour management policy can be a useful way of showing parents how children are taught socially accepted behaviour. The education of all children in this area should obviously include the exploration of feelings. Everyone has negative feelings – about themselves and others – that can be acknowledged and understood, but certain boundaries of behaviour have to be maintained for everyone's comfort and safety. A behaviour management policy should address how this is to happen.

Sample behaviour management policy

In our workplace:

1. We will always praise children whenever we can and try to reward good behaviour at all times.

2. We agree that the following types of behaviour are unacceptable
   - *All types of physical violence to another child or adult, e.g. kicking and pinching*
   - *Throwing of objects, including sand*
   - *Deliberately damaging equipment or toys*
   - *Verbal abuse of another child or adult, including remarks of a racist or sexist nature.*

3. When any such behaviour occurs, we agree that it will be dealt with using one or more of the following strategies as appropriate
   - *The child perpetrating the behaviour will be asked to stop and the reason why the behaviour is unacceptable will be explained to the child, always ensuring that the child is aware that it is the behaviour that is unacceptable, not him or her.*

- Any other child involved in the incident will be comforted and distracted as appropriate
- The perpetrator of the behaviour will be asked if they understand why their behaviour is inappropriate and will be encouraged to continue their activity in a suitable way or distracted and encouraged to do something else
- The member of staff who has dealt with the situation will keep an eye on the children and will step in quickly if the behaviour is repeated – or will inform another member of staff to do so as appropriate.

4. When any persistent behavioural problems occur and when the above strategies have not been successful in modifying the behaviour the following will be instituted:
   - Staff will meet to discuss the problem and agree on management techniques
   - The children involved will be observed to try to establish the cause of the problems and then appropriate management strategies discussed. It may be possible to remove an article of equipment that is causing persistent squabbles or to ensure that particular children are supervised when they play together.
   - In cases of extreme behaviour the child will be asked to take 'time out' in a quiet area. This will encourage and enable them to regain their composure, to recognise and reflect on their behaviour and to identify how they should behave in future – all this with the help of a supportive adult who emphasises that it is the behaviour, not the child, that is unacceptable
   - Staff will examine and discuss the activities on offer to discover whether any alteration to the layout or equipment could alleviate the problem behaviour
   - Any strategies used will be discussed and reviewed at regular intervals to identify whether they are successful, or to plan further attempts

5. All staff will:
   - Acknowledge the rights and feelings of the children and never use strategies that could humiliate the child. This includes making an example of the child, removing the right to food or drink, using a naughty chair or place
   - Undertake not to use any form of physical or emotional punishment
   - Acknowledge their own feelings and ask for another member of staff to be involved when they recognise they are not getting on with a particular child
   - Be supportive of each other and discuss strategies to ensure that children receive consistent messages about behaviour.

Further examples of Policy documents can be obtained from the Playgroup Network and Pre-school Learning Alliance. These documents provide a starting point for settings and should be amended and agreed by each individual member of the group. The policies should be regarded as working documents that are regularly updated and revised.

Evaluating a policy

All policies are working documents and, as such, should be reviewed and updated on a regular basis. The following questions may be helpful when evaluating a policy document:

1 *Does this policy cover what I want to practise in my workplace?*

2 *If not, why not?*
   - *Can it be adapted or should we start again?*
   - *Which parts are useful?*
   - *Which parts are irrelevant?*

3 *How could the policy be changed to be*
   - *Clearer?*
   - *More user friendly?*
   - *Less open to misinterpretation?*
   - *More concise?*

4 *Does the policy lend itself to practical evaluation in the workplace?*

5 *Is the policy a shared document with all members of staff taking ownership?*

Conclusion

An early years setting will need a selection of policies to document their aims and practice. Policies benefit staff by providing a unified structure for practice and are a useful source of information for parents. Staff have responsibilities to parents and children, but parents have responsibilities too. It is important that these are laid out in a clear and accessible fashion and that settings ensure that all parents have equal access to documentation.

Policies are living documents which should be reviewed and amended regularly to fit developments within the setting. The updating process can provide a forum for discussion between staff and parents. Everyone involved with the setting must take ownership of the policies and agree to abide by their provisions.

In this book we are concerned with the policies which relate particularly to children with special educational needs. These documents are the special needs policy (discussed in Chapter 3), the Welcome Booklet, the parent/carer and provider contract and the behaviour management policy.

5: MONITORING CHILDREN'S DEVELOPMENT

Key Points & Introduction

- Why monitor children's development?
- Purposes and methods of observation
- When concern should be raised
- Sample observations and assessments
- Setting targets

- How to emphasise positive achievement
- Where things can go wrong
- Ongoing monitoring and assessment
- Resources to support development.

Early years workers need an extensive knowledge of child development so that they can encourage every child to reach his or her full potential. Staff need to know what types of activities to provide to help children progress in their development, when to step in to help children move onto the next stage, and when to step back and let children find their own way. Those involved with young children need an awareness of developmental norms so that they can spot possible problems early on and intervene straight away.

However, knowledge is not enough. Early years workers must develop a repertoire of tools to help them monitor children's development. Only then can they know when individual children are making appropriate progress.

Maslow's hierarchy of needs

Everyone has needs. For example, Maslow identified needs in his pyramid diagram (Fig. 5.2) as food, shelter and safety, love and belonging, self-esteem and self-actualisation. To attain our full potential all these needs have to be met.

The theory states that, in order to reach their full potential or self-actualisation, children must fulfil the basic needs at the bottom of the triangle. Basic survival depends on children receiving food, drink and shelter. Children cannot feel safe if their need for food, drink and shelter is not fulfilled.

Equally, if a child is in an environment where they feel safe and protected their first

Figure 5.1
Maslow's hierarchy
of needs

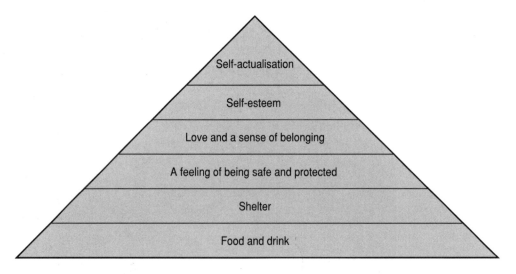

priority will not be safety. They will be able to move up the pyramid. A child who is loved and has a sense of belonging will experience the security from which self-esteem (the confidence that they are a person who is accepted and valued by others) develops. A child who does not feel loved will be more likely to have low self-esteem.

Factors influencing development

Child development is influenced by many factors. Figure 5.3 summarises these factors.

SPICE, PILES or PICES

Child development is usually broken down into the following areas:
  Physical
  Communication (language)
  Intellectual
  Social and emotional.
  These areas are know by the acronyms SPICE, PILES and PICES. Social and emotional development can also include personal and spiritual development. However development is categorised the categories interact and the sum of the parts is what makes up the whole child.

Figure 5.2

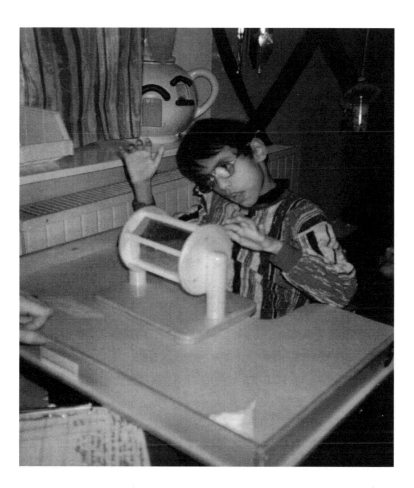

Figure 5.3
Factors influencing
children's
development

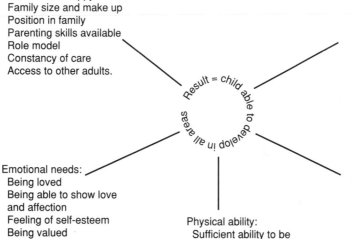

Aware of and happy with:
 Family size and make up
 Position in family
 Parenting skills available
 Role model
 Constancy of care
 Access to other adults.

Environment:
 Physical needs
 are met.

Result = child able to develop in all areas

Emotional needs:
 Being loved
 Being able to show love
 and affection
 Feeling of self-esteem
 Being valued
 Security
 Constancy of what is
 expected.

Physical ability:
 Sufficient ability to be
 able to utilise
 all or most of the
 outside influences.

Access to stimuli:
 Toys
 Books
 Materials to explore and
 experiment with
 Visual and auditory
 stimuli.

Development of children with special needs

Special needs can inhibit or delay development and, therefore, affect the potential that can be achieved. Sometimes a child's particular needs will have been apparent from birth, sometimes they will not be identified until he or she is a lot older. Any child can develop special needs as the result of illness, accident or genetic causes. Each child will have his or her own potential which is achievable and which will lead to self-actualisation. An individual child's potential will depend on the severity of their condition. A child who had an allergy to strawberries will only need to be kept away from the fruit to be able to function normally. However, a child with an inability to absorb proteins will not grow or gain strength to develop physically in the same way as his peers. Thinking back to Maslow, this child is not able to fulfil his basic nutritional needs. A lack of shelter and safety are more likely to arise when a child's social background is the inhibitor. In order to reach the top of the pyramid all the other needs must have been met. Also, the child must have received acknowledgement of their achievements and have gained an understanding that it is important to try, even if by trying there is not always an achievement – it is okay to get it wrong sometimes! Everyone makes mistakes. It is part of learning.

- A child will be unlikely to flourish if they are constantly cold, or have breathing difficulties because of damp home conditions.
- A malnourished child will not be strong physically or intellectually. She will not have developed sufficiently to question her world. She will not seek to accumulate information to utilise in her intellectual development. Finding enough to eat is her priority and leads her learning needs.
- An abused child will not feel safe. The consequence of this will also be a lack of progression in development.
- A child with sight difficulties may be unaware of the world outside his range of vision. This could affect how he is able to represent the world in terms of language and art.
- If a child is not loved or has no sense of belonging, she will not respond to social contact. She will not have a clear idea of her place in the world and will have a low opinion of herself. Behavourial problems could well be a consequence – a child who has not been given guidance may constantly test her boundaries.
- An abused child can have problems with social and emotional development. For instance, he may have difficulty building relationships involving trust. The child may be unaware of what is expected in a loving relationship without abuse.

Normative development

It is, of course, very difficult to decide what is normal development – all children are different and come with different backgrounds, experiences, needs and characters. However, it is important to be able to tell when a child is *not progressing* at an appropriate rate given their individual circumstances. Normative development has been described by many in the past and average ages and stages identified for all areas of development.

Making comparisons

How do we know when a child needs additional help? Tables of normative development detail the average age at which a child would *normally* reach a particular stage in their development. Every child follows his or her own path of individual development and will have particular areas where he or she is ahead or behind.

The average age for development of a particular skill is useful only as an *indicator*. An 'average child' walks at around their first birthday, but it is perfectly normal for a child to begin walking at 9 or 24 months without any cause for concern.

Children with special needs, as with all others, have their own developmental paths. Whilst it is useful to use normative measures to become aware of concerns about development, when a child is not achieving by normative standards it is better to record developmental advances. These may be very small advances, or substantial ones. It is important to record how the child was stimulated to achieve – at their own speed, within their own capabilities and to meet their particular needs.

Portage

One of the systems that particularly works in this way is the Portage system (see page 101). Developed in America and having been run successfully in parts of the UK for many years, this system provides encouragement through a structured programme. Very young children are able to achieve a large variety of life skills by practising a series of very small steps. These steps are agreed on a regular basis between a trained volunteer worker and the parents or carers who identify how a child is going to work towards achieving a particular goal.

This goal may take many weeks or months to achieve, but since the steps are small the child is able to achieve at their own rate. If the child is not achieving, the steps can be made easier. If the child is achieving very easily, then they can be made more difficult. Progress towards each step is methodically recorded each day by the child's parents or carers and reviewed by the carer and volunteer together.

The development of a healthy brain is affected not only by physical factors but also by mental stimulation and opportunities to explore, experience and experiment.

If a child cannot develop physically – because of a disease, condition or accident – extra care will be needed to ensure that that child has the same opportunities to develop his or her intellectual potential. Being unable to get around can limit the opportunities for exploration and, therefore, development.

Think about your own childhood. What are the memories that stand out? Do they relate to outdoor activities, trips, outings and holidays, experiences with a peer group, overcoming some obstacle, climbing a particular tree or hill? Think about how these memories would have been altered or not possible if:

- *You had some sort of physical impairment that meant some or all movement was restricted*
- *A social role model had not been available*
- *You were unable to express emotions constructively*
- *You were being abused*
- *You had had no opportunity to play with others*
- *You had no role model for clear speech*
- *There had been no resources available to you – no toys, no books, no television.*

Observation

If all children are different and they all progress at a different rate how do we identify a starting point from which to work with an individual child? How do we know when to be concerned if a particular stage of development has not been achieved? Observation is the answer. It provides a starting point telling us where a child is and what he or she might achieve. To build up a comprehensive picture of a child takes many observations. Observations have to be analysed, or assessed before judgements can be made. In the simplest form an observation might be based around a checklist like this one:

- *Can the child hold a pencil?*
- *Can he then make a mark on paper?*
- *Are the marks extended from side to side?*
- *...round and round?*
- *...up and down?*
- *Can the child make independent marks by taking the pencil on and off the paper?*
- *Can the child draw a circle?*
- *...a face?*
- *...limbs coming from the head?*
- *Does the child add a body?*
- *Does he add long limbs?*
- *Does he include digits on the limbs?*

Figure 5.4

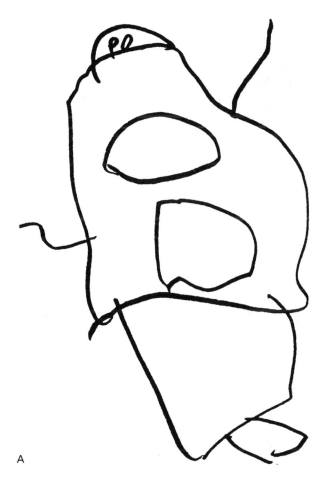

A

Figure 5.4 (*cont'd*)

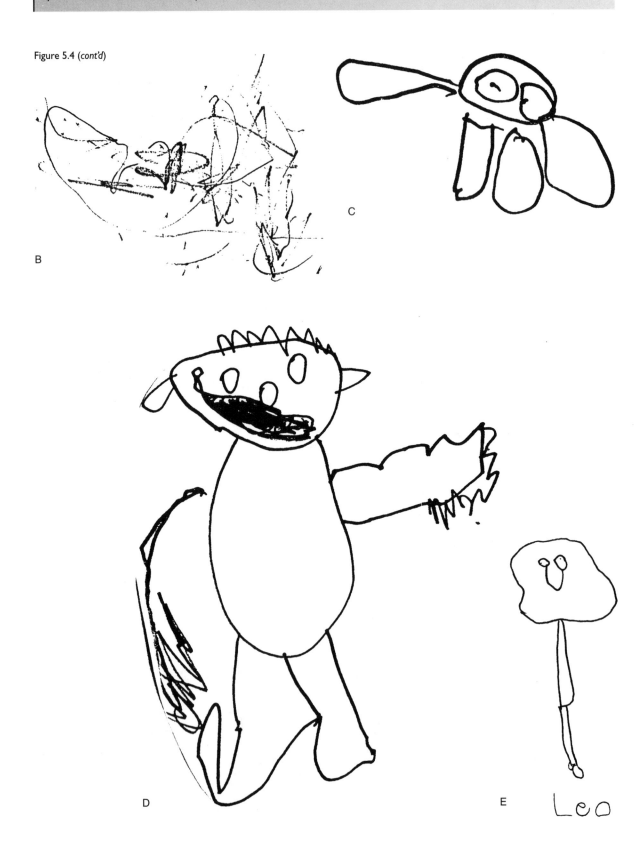

Sheila Wolfendale's work identifies a list of starting points which helps early years workers to assess the stage a particular child has reached. This enables us to draw conclusions about individual children's needs and where and how they should progress. If you know what a child's needs are you can enable the child to achieve at his or her own rate of progress rather than providing a standard programme that may not take account of his or her individual needs.

Think about where you work.

Figure 5.5
Does your workplace reflect positive images of different people?

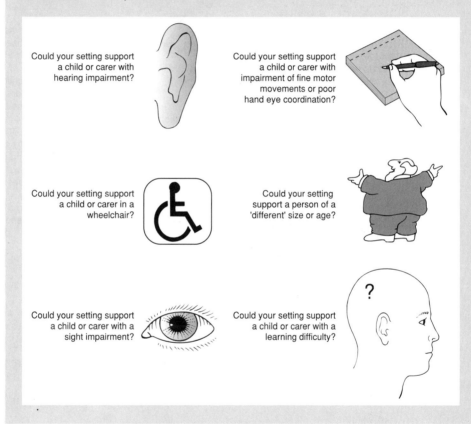

Could your setting support a child or carer with hearing impairment?

Could your setting support a child or carer with impairment of fine motor movements or poor hand eye coordination?

Could your setting support a child or carer in a wheelchair?

Could your setting support a person of a 'different' size or age?

Could your setting support a child or carer with a sight impairment?

Could your setting support a child or carer with a learning difficulty?

Methods of observation

There are many methods of observation. The starting point with all of them should be: 'What do I want to find out?' Having answered this question, you can then think about the most appropriate method of observation, the number of observations, the duration of such observations and how you will collate and utilise the information you obtain.

Before carrying out any observation you will need to obtain the permission of the

Figure 5.6
Methods of
observation

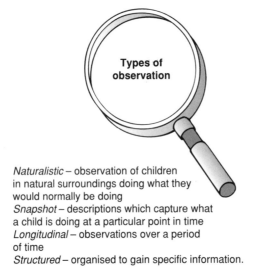

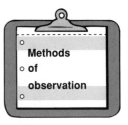

Naturalistic – observation of children in natural surroundings doing what they would normally be doing
Snapshot – descriptions which capture what a child is doing at a particular point in time
Longitudinal – observations over a period of time
Structured – organised to gain specific information.

Why observe?
* To understand children's needs
* Record development
* Identify any concerns about development
* Support a child's special needs
* To manage behaviour
* To ensure the environment meets the children's needs
* To aid planning
* Identify good practice and what needs to be changed.

Checklist of development (see page 37)
Event sampling – observing particular events
Time sampling – observing a child at regular intervals
Sociagrams – how children relate to others
Target child – specialised form of observation which focuses on one child in a group or situation
Structured records – including methods designed by educationalists
Anecdotal – recording of events as they happen
Video and audio tapes
Diaries
Tracking – recording a child's movement and activities during a period of time
Activity observation – observing an activity.

parents of the child. Talking to parents is essential and gives the early years worker an opportunity to gather pertinent information about the child and their stage of development. However, it is important to be aware of the parents' feelings. They may feel shocked or refuse to accept that there may be a problem. They will become very concerned if an early years worker insists that something is 'wrong' with their child.

Parents need to be reassured and comfortable with what is proposed for their child. They should be consulted at every stage from observation to utilisation of that information in a programme that will provide the best opportunity for their child to achieve.

Observation skills

Obviously observational skills need practice. It is very difficult, particularly with children who know you, to be the 'fly on the wall'. Just having a clipboard or something to write on, and trying to be detached will encourage the children's interest. If a child thinks you are watching them specifically, they could react in a number of ways: they may withdraw from the group, go to hide, put on an act, get very excited or completely ignore you. They may not carry on as normal because they know you are there! So, observation really is an art!

Watching and seeing

Everyone involved with children watches them constantly – to ensure their safety, that they are stimulated, behaving sociably, and most of all, that they are happy. Perhaps our starting point should be to become more aware of what our watching is actually seeing (and what we are hearing). There are clues in body language, gesture and verbal language.

To practise and hone observational skills you will need time and many opportunities to observe. If you are part of a busy workforce this may not fit easily within your role. You will need to agree with your colleagues that you need free time in which to observe. If all staff take time for observation and practise becoming detached from the group, the children will accept this as part of everyday life and observation will be easier.

Setting targets

We have discussed the need to identify a reason for observing. Try setting some targets for your observations. At first keep it simple:

- *I want to see what this child does in the next 10 minutes*
- *I want to observe who this child communicates with within the next 30 minutes*
- *I want to observe the climbing frame for 10 minutes and record the actions and language of the children using it.*

Once you have decided on what you want to observe you need to think about the best way to achieve your target. If you have a video recorder and the children are used to being filmed, this is one of the easiest methods. You can follow a particular child around and just concentrate on the operation of the camera. The children do need to be used to the camera as they must ignore it for this method to really work. Starlets may be tempted to perform whilst others will want to hide! Using our own eyes and ears can be very rewarding. Again, the biggest hurdle is getting the children to ignore you or at least to carry on as normally as possible. With time and frequent exposure, children will become familiar with the sight of you walking around watching and scribbling. Remember that you will need to be in a position where you can see and hear what is going on!

How to record?

Bearing in mind that confidentiality must be paramount, the answer to the question will depend on what you want to achieve. In all cases you need to record as much information as you can during the observation. Then go back to your original target and, using the information you have collected, ask yourself 'What have I learnt?' and then 'Is it reliable?' Was the behaviour 'typical' or not? Do you need to do the observation again? If so, should this be at a similar time, place or setting? Could you change any one of those factors to bring in more information?

Observation to identify a stage of development

Before you begin this type of observation, it may be useful to have a detailed checklist identifying the things you would expect to see in a child of comparable age. This checklist could involve very simple statements, as in the example below, or may be a weighty document running to many pages and giving very detailed and accurate information.

This chart is only suitable for observing one child at a time. For the results to be reliable, the observer would have to be sure that the test conditions were consistent for each child. For example, that the children performed the tasks at a similar time of day, with the same equipment and that a note was made and the tasks repeated if the child was unwell or was uncooperative. Whilst there is no such thing as a fair observation which takes account of *all* outside circumstances, the use of such a chart can provide a basic insight into many areas.

For individual children the chart can highlight:

- *Skills which the child has not had sufficient opportunity to practise*
- *Activities in which the child was not interested*
- *Any areas of particular achievement*
- *What the child can do.*

The chart might be used to assess the readiness of individual children to move into a reception class. Developmental areas could be loosely grouped as follows:

- *Social and emotional – activities 1, 3, 4, 5, 6, 7, 13, 17, 18, 19*
- *Physical – activities 2, 14, 15, 16, 20, 21, 22*
- *Intellectual – activities 5, 8, 11, 12, 23, 24, 25, 26, 28*

An inability to achieve, say four of the criteria in one category would not give too much cause for concern, but if there was a total lack of achievement in a category, there may be a real problem which would make it difficult for the child to cope in a classroom setting without special support.

Table 5.1   A checklist style observation form

Before starting Reception Class, the 'ideal child' can do all of the following	Tick if achieved

---

1. engage in make believe play
2. care for self at the toilet
3. share and take turns
4. enjoy playing with others
5. concentrate on activity they have chosen
6. relate appropriately to adults
7. understand the need for rules and fair play
8. name at least four colours
9. talk in sentences
10. listen attentively to stories and rhymes
11. follow simple instructions
12. recount recent events or stories in correct sequence
13. leave parent/carer without being upset
14. use scissors appropriately
15. attempt to dress and undress independently
16. copy a cross in painting/drawing
17. respond and react positively to music
18. enjoy using a range of creative materials
19. explore a 'role' through dramatic/imaginative play
20. hop, kick and stand on one leg for a short time
21. thread, build, hold a pencil correctly
22. trace over large pictures
23. knows that English script goes from left to right and top to bottom
24. recognise own name
25. sequence three pictures in logical order
26. match simple shapes
27. recite nursery rhymes
28. identify the odd one out

Observation to judge standards within a group

The chart can be used to assess the overall standard of achievement of the group. If results from the observations of the whole group are added together, it might become apparent that most of the children could not recite more than three nursery rhymes. This could be because the group has had a policy of introducing a variety of new songs to the children and only a few of the traditional rhymes have been practised.

Observations of this kind might suggest programmes of work. For example, staff might decide to concentrate on traditional rhymes, perhaps by making a large Nursery Rhyme Book with the children. However, it could be that the early years workers might feel that the children had developed the skill of listening to, learning and repeating songs and rhymes, although not in traditional forms, and that an important learning outcome had been achieved.

Observation to assess practice

The results of observations can be used to answer wide-ranging questions such as: 'Is our curriculum working?' or 'are the children achieving the skills they need to have before starting in a reception class?' or 'Do we include all children?'

Observation to assess provision

A different use of observation is to enable the observer to see how a particular activity or piece of equipment is being used by children. It is also possible to observe how a child is supported and included in the activity. The following target questions could be identified:

- *Is the activity located correctly?*
- *Are there sufficient equipment or materials?*
- *Is there sufficient space?*
- *Is there the right amount of adult interaction?*
- *Are the optimum 'number' of children using it?*
- *Is the activity more popular with girls or boys?*
- *What could be done to improve access for all children?*
- *Is the activity providing an opportunity for children to achieve any identified learning outcomes?*
- *Is the activity attractive and accessible to all children?*

Observing children with special needs

It may not be appropriate to use a standard checklist to observe a child with special needs. You must decide whether the checklist should be adapted to fit the child's needs. You need to ask yourself whether you get a better picture of the child by recording what they can do, rather than what they can't.

One answer to this dilemma might be to write a purely narrative report, describing the child as a whole. Another method might be to use the criteria listed in the checklist and to comment on (rather than just tick) the child's achievements. For example:
15. Can dress and undress unaided:

Peter can dress and undress himself. However he has only limited use of one hand and needs extra time to do so. This statement identifies both achievement and need.

Both of the methods outlined above would provide information about the child's achievements, rather than lack of them, but would not provide a context for comparison with his or her peers.

The Code of Practice

The table below is intended to give an overall picture of how observation should be used in line with the Code of Practice requirements. Chapter 3 deals with the Code in some detail.

Table 5.2 Observation and the Code of Practice

Stage 1
- *General observations as part of normal settling in practice, incorporating the view of parents*
- *Note made of any concerns based on evidence collected*
- *Concerns may be short term*
  Record concerns on special needs register.

Stage 2
Review of Stage 1
- *Note which strategies assist learning*
- *Note rate of progress*
- *Set targets within normal curriculum*
- *Involve parents*
- *Prepare Individual Education Plan and monitor progress.*

Stage 3
Review of Stage 2
- *Use specialised observation and assessment strategies*

Table 5.2 (cont'd)

- *More emphasis on norm referenced assessment*
- *Parents and other professionals involved*
- *Monitor progress in relation to Individual Education Plan.*

Stage 4

Review of Stage 3

- *Formal assessment*
- *Individual multi-disciplinary assessment*
- *Involve parents fully*
- *Results of Individual Education Plan taken into account.*

Stage 5

Review

- *Formal record of progress and provision*
- *Individual Education Plan becomes part of ongoing review.*

Using comparative charts

Another method of identifying the norms of developmental achievement is to use a comparative chart. An example is shown in Figure 5.7.

The comparative chart shows the very wide range that can be regarded as 'normal' development in this particular area. It shows potentially very able children at one end of the spectrum and those with possible problems at the other.

Able children

Early achievers have very specific needs. They may not be advanced in every stage of development. Whilst it might be very tempting to place a child with exceptional intellectual prowess with older children who are on the same level intellectually, the child may not be matched in other ways. He will not be the same size physically, he may not have the same level of personal and interpersonal skills. Such a placement would be inappropriate to meet the needs of the whole child. However, it is equally inappropriate to place able children with their age peers if they are presented with a level of work which they do not find challenging. There is a risk of developing unacceptable behaviour through frustration and lack of stimulation. Once again, we return to the fact that it is important to look at the child *holistically* and to provide for their individual needs in all areas.

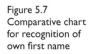

Figure 5.7
Comparative chart
for recognition of
own first name

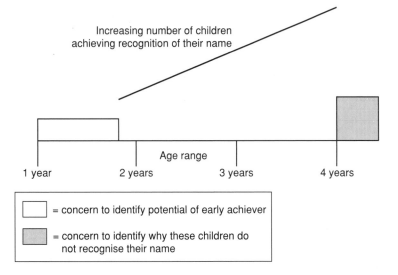

Increasing number of children
achieving recognition of their name

Age range

1 year   2 years   3 years   4 years

□ = concern to identify potential of early achiever

▨ = concern to identify why these children do
    not recognise their name

Sample observation and assessments

The following pages show five sample observation and assessments of real children gathered in real settings. Names and details have been changed to protect the children's identities. Different methods were used according to circumstances and the objectives for the observations:

> *Sample 1 is an activity observation*
> *Sample 2 is a narrative child observation focussing on what the child does*
> *Sample 3 is a narrative child observation focussing on what the child says*
> *Sample 4 is a tracking observation*
> *Sample 5 is a time sampling observation.*

Sample observation and assessment 1
CONFIDENTIAL

- *Setting: Four children (J, K, L and M), all boys, playing with a variety of LEGO bricks. They are all just approaching their fourth birthdays.*
- *Purpose: To observe a specific activity and assess how it is being used.*
- *Date: 4.5.1999*
- *Time: 10.30 am*
- *Place: Preschool Group*
- *Permission: Parental permission obtained*

Table 5.3	Activity Observation		
	What are the children doing? What role is the adult taking?	**How many girls and boys?**	**What is being said?**
At the start	K, L and M are talking about their holidays – pool. Adult is at the table just listening. M selects the largest board he can find. M, K and L sort through and find all the blue bricks, J watches for a minute or two and then also starts collecting blue bricks. They all add them to the edge of the board – M going right along one side, K building up in a stepped pile and L, building along and up a shorter side. J places the bricks more slowly and without any apparent meaningful pattern.	4 boys	K < I swam in the hotel. L < So did I. M <Me, too – shall we make a pool together? Adult < J Did you go swimming too? J nods. M <Our pool had a blue bottom – let's find all the blue bricks. K < I building the steps down. L < I'm building the diving board.
After 5 minutes	The boys have built the various sides up to different levels. J side has bricks in different lines. M, K and L continue to build.		M<J You haven't got yours straight – let me help – you find some more bricks. Adult < J I'll help you find some more blue bricks shall I? J nods.
After 10 minutes	K gets up and leaves the table, L joins him. M continues to build, J is sitting watching the two departing boys.		K<L I've have enough of this – let's play with the sand! M < Adult I want to finish it – will you help me? J nods.

Table 5.3 (cont'd)	Activity Observation		
	What are the children doing? What role is the adult taking?	**How many girls and boys?**	**What is being said?**
After 15 minutes	M and the Adult have now built a four sided construction and are building up the diving board. J is joining in spasmodically.	2 boys	A< M and J Where did you go on holiday? M < Adult We went to Spain – it was great! A<J Where did you go J? J<A The beach A<J Can you remember where the beach was? J shakes his head.

- Was the activity used by one sex more than the other?
  In this case there were only boys using the activity but I did notice during the morning some girls joined in, but not for long.
- Were the children doing what you expected?
  I was surprised that the children decided on such a definite task. They were encouraged by the adult but two of them lost interest after a while. One child maintained interest for a long time. I have concerns about J's level of participation, language and comprehension and will carry out further observations to find out if this behaviour is normal for him or whether there is a specific cause today. Although he followed and stuck with the activity, he seemed to be doing it because it was expected of him, rather than any real desire to complete the task. He showed no initiative or input into the activity.
- What was the role played by any adults involved? Was it appropriate?
  I felt the adult role in this case was very supportive and encouraging. She was asking appropriate questions and being encouraging without taking over the activity and directing the children.
- Did the activity promote language?
  Yes, the children talked amongst themselves and to the adult utilising outside experiences.
- What skills or development was the activity encouraging?
  Manipulative skills, problem-solving and reasoning, colour recognition.

Sample observation and assessment 2
CONFIDENTIAL
Child's Initials: DG
Sex: female
Age: 3 years 6 months
Date: 28.9.99
Time from: 10.00
to: 10.15
Place: Playgroup
Permission: Parental permission given

Why is this observation being carried out?   D started playgroup immediately after her third birthday and was lively and interested in all she did. Since she rejoined the group at the beginning of September she seems to be not paying attention to anyone, playing alone, and has lost a lot of her interest in activities.

Description of setting   There is a wide range of activities set up including: domestic play area, painting easel, drawing table with mirrors for children to draw their own pass-port photos, collage materials relating to theme of holidays, Travel Agents desk and a wide range of books and posters for discussion with adult. A group of chairs are set out as an aeroplane with boxes that have been decorated for the flight deck. A very large box has been turned into a ferry, and further chairs are set up to represent a train and coach with relevant props. The sand tray has various forms of transport in it to encourage talk about what will move in sand and what won't. The water tray is next to a table with a variety of materials to test sinking/floating and to make boats. The boats will be constructed with the children and then tested to see if they float and move by blowing or agitating the water. The results will be recorded on a simple pictorial chart to indicate which one floated the longest – an adult will support this activity. The book corner is set out with a large variety of books and the 'today shelf' displays lots of books showing transport and foreign countries. A cooking activity – making croissants is just beginning. Dressing up clothes providing a range of ethnic costumes are available to the children. Three adults are in the room, all deployed on a general basis.

Observation (narrative of what happened over period of observation)   D is sitting on the bottom step of the stage, cradling a doll in her arms and watching the cooking activity. She is invited to join by the adult but does not respond. The adult approaches her and asks again if she would like to join in, indicating a free seat at the table. D nods, drops the doll and runs to sit down. The adult asks her to pick up the doll and wash her hands before cooking. D half turns and then turns back to the table. The adult picks up the doll and sits it on the steps. She returns to the table and reminds all the children that they must wash their hands before beginning. Two boys get up and go towards the washing bowl, D follows. The other two girls show their hands and say they have washed them. D returns to the table and watches the adult getting out the ingredients and talking about them. She tells the children they are to make croissants and asks them to repeat the word. D does not join in. The adult then explains that croissants are often eaten in France at breakfast time and asks each child what they had for breakfast. When asked directly D shakes her head. The adult then asks if she did not have breakfast, again D shakes her head. The adult suggests that D may have eaten a cereal for breakfast and when she goes through a list, D nods when she gets to Weetabix. The adult gets out the scales and points to the numbers. She then asks each child to identify an ingredient and pour in sufficient to reach the required quantity on the scales. D is asked to begin and given the flour. She says flour when asked what it is and pours in enough until it reaches when the adult indicated. The activity progresses with the other children and D watches intently and joins in with the mixing when the bowl is passed to her. When the activity is over she follows the others to wash her hands and then returns to the steps and picks up her doll. She puts her thumb in her mouth and watches the group.

Interpretation   This child seemed very capable of following instructions and completing a task, but did not always comply when spoken to. She showed good dexterous skills when handling the ingredients, and knew the correct noun for flour. She was quieter than her peers and did not join in their general chatter.

Evaluation   Specific changes have been noted in this child's behaviour. These were seen during the observation and I have concerns as to whether she was hearing properly. She did not show any sign of not *wishing* to comply with instructions. The most likely explanation for not picking up the doll when asked to, was that she did not hear. I will try out various other observations and actions e.g. speaking to her from behind, asking her parents/carers if she has had a cold or ear infection that may be causing a temporary problem. I would advise that regular observations be carried out to monitor D's hearing and to advise her parents to consult a doctor if she continues to show signs of not hearing.

Whilst a hearing difficulty would appear to be a possible cause of this child's change in behaviour, other causes should not be ruled out. Continued observation is essential to gain further data.

Sample observation and assessment 3

CONFIDENTIAL

Child's Initials: KI

Sex: male

Age: 3 years 10 months

Date: 11.9.99

Time from: 10.30

to: 10.40

Place: Preschool

Permission: Yes

Why is this observation being carried out?   K has always shown a keen interest in cars and seems very bright. The object of this observation will be twofold – firstly to identify if the activities on offer stimulate the child and also to assess his vocabulary and understanding of language. Being K's keyworker, I must be aware of using my observational skills without being influenced by my background knowledge of the child. I plan to sit with him and engage him in conversation (usually very easily done).

Description of setting   There is a wide range of activities set up including: domestic play area, painting easel, drawing table. A collection of child-sized chairs have been put in one place, some have steering wheels attached to them. Children can make up their own cars, lorries, buses etc. using a number of chairs. They are encouraged to think about what the whole of their car would look like and to represent this in a painting or drawing. The sand tray has various forms of transport in it, together with road-making vehicles and materials. The children are encouraged to make roads and, if possible, a bridge strong enough to support a toy car. The water tray has a car ferry and some cars. The children are to see how many cars the ferry will take without sinking! The book corner is set out with a large variety of books and the 'today shelf' displays lots of books about road transport. A cooking activity – supported by an adult – is making traffic light biscuits. The group has collected a large number of glossy magazines showing cars. The children can cut and stick pictures onto paper and design a number plate for their vehicle. There are also car 'jigsaws' made from manufacturers' pictures of cars cut into three pieces – the children can then make up a complete car by choosing three relevant sections. There are also pictures of engines and other accessories that they can add to their pictures as they wish.

Observation

A<Hello K, How are you today?

K<I'm fine, do you want me?

A<I was wondering if you would like to make up a picture of your ideal car. There are lots of bits and pieces here. While you are doing it I would like to talk to you and write down some notes. I will use my notes to help us plan activities that you all like, and alter activities that you don't like. Is that alright with you?

K< Okay. [K sits at the table and selects a large piece of sugar paper, bright orange.] Where are the car pieces? Oh I see them. [He pulls the three boxes of main pieces of car towards him and looks through them. K selects a very sporty front in red.]

I like this one.

A<K Why do you like it K?

K< It looks like it would go very fast and it's got alloy wheels. [He proceeds to stick the selected picture to the left-hand edge of the paper so that the car front is nearest to the left hand side of the paper.] I need a middle bit now. [He selects the middle section of a large saloon car.] This one has plenty of room for me and my brothers!

A<K Do you think it will fit with the front you have chosen?

K<A Yes, it could be welded on!

A<K How would they do that?

K<A They have big drill things that get very hot and melt the metal together. [K sticks the middle piece of car on his paper, positioning it so that the wheels are more or less level. He looks at the picture.] This bit [the middle] is a lot higher than the front – we could have another windscreen and then Jake, Li and I could look through it – that would be great!

A<K Can you find a picture of a windscreen? [K looks through the accessories pile but does not find what he wants.] Perhaps you could cut one from one of the car bits. [K looks through the car fronts and selects a van screen. He then cuts it out using the scissors correctly and sticks it in the appropriate place.]

K<A There, all I need now is a boot. [He looks through the pile of backs and selects the back of a large estate car.] Plenty of room in here – my dog would like that!

A<K What's your dog's name K?

K<A He's called Dino and he's a red setter. Mum says he's mad like us! [He laughs.]

A<K Why is he mad K?

K<A He races round in circles chasing his tail and sometimes he chases other dogs and doesn't come back when he is called.

A<K Do you chase your tail?

K<A No silly, I haven't got one! If I had I'd like one like the monkey I saw in the zoo – he used his to swing on!

A<K What else did you see at the zoo K?

K<A Lots, we drove through some of it – an elephant came right past us, but the lions were lazy and asleep, we could only just see them. The monkeys were great fun – they jumped all over the car in front of us. Dad said he was glad they weren't on ours, but I would have liked that!

A<K Did you like the monkeys best K?

K<A No, I liked the sea lions – we fed them from a boat – it was very smelly though! Have I finished this picture now? [He had stuck the remaining piece on the back and was idly looking at the accessories.]

A<K It's up to you, do you want to add anything else to it?

K<A I like these lights – my dad has good fog lights – he flashes them when we get home so mum knows we're coming. [He cuts the lights from the picture and sticks them over the original lights on the front of the car.]

A<K Is there anything else you'd like?

K<A It would need a good engine, but you can't see that with the bonnet down, so I think I've finished.

A<K Would you like to put the picture to dry then? [K nods and takes the picture over to the drier.]

Interpretation

K was interested in the activity, but did not focus his whole attention on it. He was happy and very able to converse about related subjects. This child seems to be very able and we need to ensure that activities on offer do stretch him. He needs access to adult conversation, both in small groups and one-to-one, to ensure that his needs are being met.

Evaluation

The activity worked well with this child. It will be interesting to see feedback from other staff to find out whether other children found it suitable and enjoyable. K has a very good grasp of concepts of size and was able to point out easily where things didn't fit. His overall vocabulary was very good and his sentence forming was clear and accurate. He has a lively sense of humour. K showed excellent fine motor skills with the scissors. He didn't use any colours during his speech. I will set up an activity using colours to check his knowledge.

Sample observation and assessment 4

The following example identifies how a child moves around and describes briefly what they do. This is a tracking observation. This type of observation is very visual but not designed to produce as much detailed information as some of the other methods.

Figure 5.8
Tracking observation

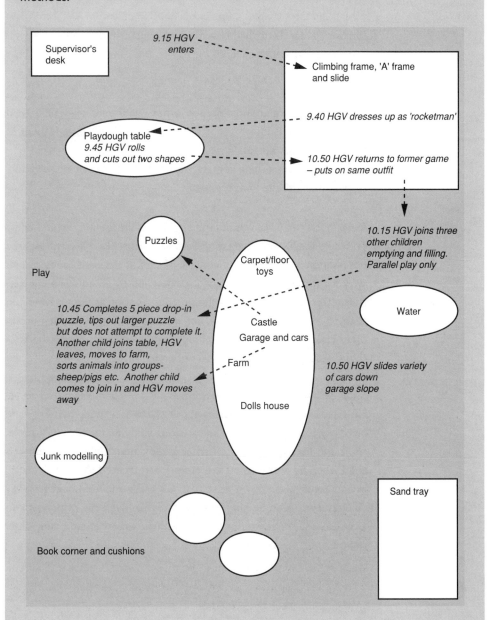

Supervisor's desk

9.15 HGV enters

Climbing frame, 'A' frame and slide

9.40 HGV dresses up as 'rocketman'

Playdough table
9.45 HGV rolls and cuts out two shapes

10.50 HGV returns to former game – puts on same outfit

10.15 HGV joins three other children emptying and filling. Parallel play only

Puzzles

Play

Carpet/floor toys

10.45 Completes 5 piece drop-in puzzle, tips out larger puzzle but does not attempt to complete it. Another child joins table, HGV leaves, moves to farm, sorts animals into groups-sheep/pigs etc. Another child comes to join in and HGV moves away

Castle
Garage and cars

Farm

Water

10.50 HGV slides variety of cars down garage slope

Dolls house

Junk modelling

Sand tray

Book corner and cushions

Child's initials: HGV
Age: 2 years 2 months
Place: Under Fives Group
Time from: 9.15
to: 10.50 am

Purpose: To identify if child is settling into group and whether he makes any attempt at socialising with other children.

Conclusion
Child does not seem interested in other children at present time, mainly involved in solitary play. He is interested in activities and will investigate them. Is capable of some parallel play and accepts that group has large number of children although not yet interested in establishing contact with peers. Will repeat observation in one month to see whether situation has changed.

A month later the child was observed again and the following conclusion was drawn.
This child is still not progressing beyond solitary play. He has been observed during this observation and by other members of staff at different times making an effort to get away from other children. When approached by an adult he will stand and listen, but tries to remove himself from the situation as soon as possible. He continues to be very keen to explore the activities, but does stick to those which are not being used by other children. He avoids role play, even when encouraged by the key worker to join in. Observations to be increased to once a fortnight.

A specific activity observation was carried out on HGV during a craft session.
He seems to really like stories about space and the activity on offer was to make a night sky using black paper and various shiny materials. HGV sat down opposite an adult and listened to her when she explained the activity. He scowled at another child when he approached the table. He retreated. A second child also tried to join in and actually sat down next to HGV. HGV moved his chair away from the other child and scowled at him. The child then moved his chair away from HGV's. They worked beside each other for some minutes. When an adult joined the table HGV ran off.

Sample observation and assessment 5

CONFIDENTIAL

Child's initials: KO [female]

Age: 3 years 2 months

Setting: Nursery

Parental permission: Yes

Reason for observation: Concerns about behaviour – aggression shown to other children.

Plan: To record incidents of bad behaviour as they happen – if possible with antecedents.

Evaluation: To be shared and discussed with other members of staff.

Table 5.4 Time sampling observation

Time	Record of behaviour
9.05	G reported that K pushed him out of the way in the corridor after hanging up their coats. K said G pushed her first. Both children then tried to push each other again. Two adults took the children separately and talked to them. G was adamant that he hadn't done anything, K sulked, thumb in mouth, turned head from adult and wouldn't respond. Adult suggested K came to listen to a story with two other children.
9.15	K pushed another child as they were getting up from story time. The other child was immediately in front of her. K said sorry when child turned round. Adult reinforced that it is unacceptable to push and that K should make sure she does not move if someone is in her way. She should wait until they move or ask them to move.
9.25	K playing with the water with two other children, one boy, one girl. The boy described how his brother could dive into the water and demonstrated using plastic figure causing a large splash as he did so. K then dived her arm into the water causing a large amount to spill out. All three children ended up with very wet feet! Adult approached K and told her that was not a suitable way to play and that she should come and sit down to complete a craft activity. Another adult took the two other children and changed their socks and shoes.
9.40	K had been sitting watching the craft activity, but not joining in. The adult suggested a starting point for her – to draw a very simple pattern, or shapes to be filled in with a variety of collage materials. K took a pencil and scribbled a line. She then took the pot of glue, emptied quite a lot on the paper, selected some rice and put a pile on top. She said, 'There!' to the adult and walked off.
9.45	Adult went after K and suggested that she should have some time out by sitting with the adult and watching what was going on. K shook her head and walked away. The adult went to restrain her and K bit her arm.

Conclusions

K's behaviour was not acceptable. Various questions should be asked: Why does the behaviour occur? Is it a pattern? Does the child think that she is perceived as bad and therefore should behave like this? Were the activities offered to the child appropriate? Was the adult interaction appropriate? Had any adult built a relationship with this child? Were the adults inadvertently using negative body language with this child? Was she aware of being treated differently to the other children? (NB: she remained in wet socks and shoes – the others changed.)

An overall strategy should be developed with the staff of the group and a behaviour management plan developed. This should be reviewed regularly. The adults should make a conscious effort to get to know this child and encourage her to become more sociable with her peers, perhaps introducing one other child at a time. As she already seems to have established a pattern of behaviour, perhaps the child could attend different sessions to enable a new start. Consultation with her parents is essential. Is there any reason why this behaviour should be happening? Have there been any changes in home life or circumstances? How do her parents find her behaviour at home etc.?

Behaviour management programme
Name of child: KO

List of Strengths

K is beginning to show signs of social play and usually conforms to the wishes of an adult.

List of Concerns

Aggression to other children and adults. Lack of interest in activities presented and does not appear to participate in activities or enjoy them.

Priority Concern

To stop aggression, ensure an understanding of why acceptable behaviour is necessary and bring about participation in activities.

To integrate child into group and break cycle of unacceptable behaviour.

Strategy to be Used

Parents to be consulted and joint strategy agreed. Suggest one-to-one work with child, ensuring praise used whenever possible. Talk to child about what is acceptable behaviour and why it is important. Accentuate this on all occasions. Identify unacceptable behaviour instantly. Explain why it is unacceptable and what behaviour would have been appropriate in the circumstances. Encourage child to identify why she behaved in the way that she did and ask her to identify alternative behaviours. Ask her to judge whether they would have been acceptable or not, and why. Reinforce group rules on behaviour during every session using positive approach. Whole group to be asked, 'What is our rule about ... (for example, throwing sand)?' Reinforce this with, 'Why do we have this rule?'

Ensure child knows what activities are on offer and try to discover her likes and dislikes. Work at providing activities she finds interesting and stimulating. Build up her confidence and encourage her to make positive choices.

Rewards

Lots of praise and encouragement. Positive body language, smiles. Free choice of activities.

Records

Desired behaviour will be recorded as part of general assessment process. Also daily report to parents of achievements. If feedback to parents is negative, or a discussion is necessary, this should take place without child present.

Date Started	*Date for Review*
21.3.00	28.3.00 at staff team meeting

Activity

The behaviour problem outlined above could have arisen for a number of reasons, some of which are suggested here:

- *The child was not introduced to the group's behaviour policy in a positive way*
- *The child did not understand the policy*
- *Staff did not make the requirements clear*

- Behaviour requirements at the nursery were not agreed with, understood or reinforced by parents
- The child has not reached a stage in her development where she can cope with these expectations
- The child did not know what to expect from nursery
- There was a lack of socialisation with other children
- There was no role model at home
- There was a physical cause such as poor hearing
- The child was put off by something that happened early on – perhaps aggressive behaviour by another child, which she perceived as being the norm of behaviour.

The danger, if this situation were to continue, would be that the child would be labelled as uncooperative or out of control. The child would become aware of the way she was perceived and would reflect that in her behaviour – I'm expected to misbehave therefore I shall! Her self-esteem would be greatly diminished leading to a loss of interest in learning, which could continue in a downward spiral.

Think about the whole situation. What is your personal interpretation of it? What would you do in this case? Do you agree with the Behaviour Management Plan?

Using observation to inform planning

As we become more competent in our observational techniques, the aims of our observations can become more specific and increasingly targeted to what we wish to find out. For example, when observing a child with unclear speech, we could tick a column on our observation sheet every time the child uses one double consonant correctly and tick another column for a sound that is not being said correctly. To take this observation into the planning stage we would arrange activities, such as games, stories and conversations, that involve the difficult sound.

Once we have used our observational skills to assess a child's developmental stage we can identify a starting point and targets to aim for.

We need as much information as possible on each child as an individual to assess:

- What will be the next stage in their development in any particular area
- How best to encourage progress – the steps along the way
- What resources, parent and staff support are needed to achieve this
- How and when review will take place.

Case Study

Observation can be used to evaluate activities to ensure that what was planned actually happened and that the needs of all the children were met. This is an example of a planned activity which was evaluated by observation. The specific focus was how a child with special educational needs was included and a ten minute observation during the activity targeted this child.

The following remit was given to a classroom assistant:

Please plan a Reception Class session including a description of what activities and equipment you would put out to promote the theme of 'Safety at School' to the children. Give details of a display you would put together with them to illustrate this theme. Include an interest table as part of this display and give examples of what could be included. Such items would either be available from the school or the children will be asked to bring in items from home. Describe any adaptations or alterations you would make to your plans to ensure you meet the needs of Mina who recently started with us and has 50% sight loss.

This is the assistant's plan:

1. Initial discussion session with the children to plan display and interest table. Introduce subject of safety and ask children to accompany me around the building and playground whilst I record areas where we need to be aware of safety issues: general access to the school, fences and boundaries, plants and trees including poisonous varieties, access doors, flooring surfaces, fire exits, cloakroom area (check for things left lying about), storage of equipment. I would take notes and also ask the children to draw, make notes and, if possible, take photographs. During this exercise, my one specific concern for Mina would be to ensure that she stayed to the front of the group, and perhaps had a magnifying glass with her. All the children could use this for looking at details of plants.
2. We would follow this exercise by producing a large display of our findings. The children would be asked to paint in the background and then add their pictures, notes and photos. We would discuss an appropriate title for the display and I suggest that we think about using ribbons – luminous coloured paper strips – which would lead to a set of safety rules.
3. Our interest table – to go under the display – could have examples of safety features, e.g. clothing with fluorescent patches and pictures of safety equipment such as fire extinguishers, a fire blanket, a picture of the class carrying out a fire drill.

4. The subject could be extended by asking the children to think, draw and write about safety in other contexts – at home, on the way to school, out shopping.

5. The display would stay up for about two weeks and during this period it would be referred to in general class activities so that the children's understanding and increased safety awareness can develop and be assessed.

Mina would be able to join in all the above activities. If possible, her increased awareness of other senses could be highlighted to show that children could use all their senses to be aware of possible dangers – particularly listening as well as looking when going round a corner, for example.

A student observed an activity which was part of the 'safety at school' theme. Here is her record:

Setting: The practical area is set out with a large roll of frieze paper unrolled. There is another table with various bits and pieces collected during the health and safety survey carried out yesterday. Also available are a wide range of collage materials, paints and different types of paper. Everyone is wearing a plastic apron. Present at the table – classroom assistant [CA], Ben [B], Luke [L], Irene [I] and Mina [M]. The student's role as an observer has been explained to the children and they have been asked to ignore her.

Date: 21.8.99   Time from: 10.00 am   To: 10.15 am   Place: Infant school

Table 5.5   Student observation

Activity	Language
The CA welcomes the children and explains the task before them. She asks if anyone has any ideas about where they should start.	B< Let's paint a big picture with lots of people having accidents – they would see all the blood and stop doing silly things! CA< That's an interesting idea Ben, but what about helping people think of all the right things to do so they don't have accidents in the first place? B<I'd rather see the blood! CA <What does everyone else think? I<I don't like blood, Yuk! M<I think we should show people what the danger is and tell them what to do – like crossing the road – things we should remember. CA<That's a very good idea – what about if we paint pictures of the school – outside, the

---

Table 5.5 *(cont'd)*

Activity	Language
	playground, and inside. Then we could stick all the things we collected on it and at the end put a list of safety rules.
The children all nod.	CA<Right, who would like to paint the school? B<I will – can it be red? L<No silly our school's not painted red – no one would know what it was supposed to be! CA<What colour is the outside of the school Ben? B<Sort of grey, but it's not all the same. CA<Yes that's right. Why don't you have a go at mixing the colours until you get a brick colour? B<Okay.
B moves over to paints and begins to mix up colours in a palette.	CA<Irene what do you want to paint? I<I'd like to do the corridor – the floor's like hopscotch! CA<Off you go then.
L moves to the collage table and selects the sand.	L<I'm going to make the pit we jump in. CA<Yes, Luke but where is the pit? L<At the end of the field, just before the fence. CA<Yes so perhaps we could ask Mina to paint the fence in so you know where to put the sand? M<It should go at one end – which end?
CA looks at the paper and points to the right-hand end. Mina selects some black paint, a medium brush and starts to paint a long line onto the paper. B indicates with his brush.	M<How long should the fence be? CA<Let's think – when we walked through the playground we timed that it took twice as long as walking through the school – so we said we thought that must mean that the playground was twice as long. B<Where are you putting the school wall? CA<Mina that's Ben's end of the wall [she puts her hand to also indicate place] I think you should finish the fence here – is that OK? M<Yes.
M puts a large black dot to indicate the end of the fence and goes back to the other end to paint lines to indicate the fence.	

To see if the observation served its purpose, the questions to ask would be:

> - *Were the aims and objectives of the plan achieved?*
> - *Was the interaction between the adult and children appropriate?*
> - *Were Mina's needs being met?*
> - *Were the needs of the other children being met?*
> - *If there was anything that could have been changed about the activity, what was it and why?*

Objectivity when observing

Consider the following extract which is taken from an observation of a child who seemed to have behavioural problems.

Reason for observation

PL has not settled into the school since he started last January. He is disruptive and uninterested in any of the activities, preferring to institute fights and squabbles.

Description of setting

The classroom is set out to provide activities for a group of 20 children ranging in age from 3 to 4 years. At one table there is a craft activity where the classroom assistant is seated directing the production of Easter cards – working with a group of four children at a time. There is a choice of either a chick or rabbit in yellow, pink or blue. Pre-cut pieces are stuck on the front of the card and the children are asked to add eyes, beaks, feet, whiskers and other features as appropriate. Another group are sitting building a LEGO construction which is a continuing activity from the previous day. Books are set out attractively in a corner, complete with cushions and chairs. Another table has a variety of puzzles and a further table has fuzzy felts set out on it. The teacher is working with three children to complete a display of daffodils that have been made previously and are being added to a spring garden that runs the length of one wall.

Observation

PL had been looking at books for about 10 minutes and now gets up and wanders around. The teacher asks him if he would like to join in with the group making the display. PL shakes his head. He goes over to the card activity and sits down next to another child. The boy says, 'Go away P – you spoil our games!' P says, 'No I don't – you are silly' and he pushes the boy. The boy pushes him back and then P punches him. By this time the teacher has arrived and takes P by the hand. She says, 'You know we don't fight – now I want you both to say "sorry" to each other.' Both boys mumble an apology. The teacher says, 'P you will now please come with me.' P follows her back to the wall display. The other children move away from him as he comes up and he scowls at them. The teacher says, 'Let's finish our garden – I think it looks lovely – what flowers do you like best H?' H replies, 'I likes the crocuses.' The teacher turns back to the wall and continues to stick on daffodils which H and J are passing to her. O and N are sticking leaves to some more daffodils before they go on the wall. P stands and watches them all. O sticks the glue brush on his hand. P yelps and takes the brush from O and throws it on the floor. The teacher turns round and says to O, 'Please pick up the brush and finish what you are doing. P if you can't join in with us, you will have to sit by yourself over there.' She points to a chair which is away from everyone else. P walks over and sits down. After a couple of minutes he is rocking the chair. The teacher tells him to stop. The classroom assistant has a space at the table and calls P over to make his card. P sits down and takes a card. He selects the pieces for a rabbit and begins to stick them on. The class assistant says, 'Please wait P I haven't told you what to do yet.' She then turns back to the child she was working with and continues her explanation. P sticks his rabbit together and adds eyes, a mouth, nose, whiskers and lines for inner ears. He also draws in paws. He gets up to go. The class assistant asks him to wait. He sits down again. After a couple of minutes P takes the glue brush and starts to make a pattern with the glue on the newspaper. The class assistant says, 'Stop making a mess P, I'll be with you in a minute.' P sits and swings his legs, kicking the underside of the table with increasing force so that the things on the table jog up and down. The class assistant says, 'You are being impossible this morning P – go back to your chair.' P returns to the chair and immediately starts to rock the chair. He gets faster and faster until the chair tips over. The teacher then comes over again.

Evaluation

This child seems incapable of occupying himself in a positive way and responds to others in a very negative way. He is also aggressive, although this is usually in response to others. His reactions are inappropriate given the level of aggression shown to him. He has built up a pattern of poor behaviour with the other children in the group. I would recommend that this child be considered for referral for specialist help.

The above observation, although accurate, was undertaken by someone who had been working very closely with this child, and who had come to expect that he would behave badly. The interpretation of the observation is not objective and various factors have not been taken into account. The staff team have been used to working with five-year-olds prior to this and are not experienced in working with this age group.

This child has been singled out and labelled. He is behaving badly because he is expected to behave in this way. The management of his behaviour has not tackled the reason for it at all.

Let's now look at the above scenario from the child's point of view. He is a very bright little boy, keen to have new experiences. He excels at physical activities and is used to lots of adult input at home. He is taken care of by his grandfather after school and they are both very interested in transport. His grandfather is an expert at making mechanical models which they test out together. Remote control cars are amongst their favourites, although they also have model boats, and a railway layout. P feels constantly got at at school. He is also bored and frustrated most of the time. Being unused to the company of his peers, he does not know how to socialise with them and they, sensing his insecurity, tease and torment him. He responds with aggression. If this situation was allowed to continue his self-esteem would be affected and he is already beginning to see himself in a negative way. This child's needs are not being met within this setting. There is a very real danger of his label sticking and his behaviour becoming worse. It is likely that observations will continue to concentrate on the negative aspects of his behaviour and staff will come to see him only as a nuisance.

This case highlights the effects of bringing our personal backgrounds, working situation and feelings into interpretation of observations. We need to observe accurately – just what we see, rather than what we *think* we see. The evaluation or interpretation of our observations must be objective. We should try to balance our personal feelings by asking the question: 'How else could this be interpreted?'

Critical incident analysis

The use of critical incident analysis when working with children can help to identify a starting point for planning. In this form of analysis we ask: What can the child do? What does the child enjoy? What can be provided to stimulate their progression?

Case Study

Peony had been observed by her parents and playgroup workers over a period of 6 months following concern over her communication skills. At nearly 4 years of age she was not forming sentences and her vocabulary was not developing. Her hearing had been checked out and was found to be slightly deficient in one ear. Medical intervention was not necessary. Peony could make a range of sounds but had developed her own language which she used when playing by herself. Peony was an only child. Her parents both liked classical music and spending time quietly at home. They did not have a television. There were no other relations living close by.

Peony was still at the stage of solitary play. She was quite happy to watch the other children, but did make any attempt to join in their games or become part of the group. She would join in with a group when asked to do so, but would slip away as soon as possible and go back to playing on her own. She particularly liked playing with small world figures and equipment, and also liked the dolls' house, farm and zoo. She would manipulate the various figures and act out stories for herself. She enjoyed listening to music, but not so much to stories, although if there were lots of pictures she showed more interest. When playing matching games she was able to select objects when asked and put two pictures together, but did not repeat the words.

It was decided that this was a very specific type of language delay and that Peony should receive some individual attention to try to increase her communication skills. Staff and Peony's parents decided that they would build on Peony's interests with activities at nursery and at home. Peony was on a waiting list to see a speech therapist but the first appointment was not for another 3 months. An important point was that Peony would be praised at every opportunity.

Strategy 1
Peony's keyworker would spend some time with her individually, trying to join in her games. The group had purchased a new set of Sylvannian families figures. These would be 'introduced' by the keyworker who would use their names. She would then initiate a story and ask Peony to take up the narrative at an appropriate moment. The keyworker would continue to tell the story following and interpreting Peony's movements and asking her frequently if she was getting the story right. These particular figures would only be used when the keyworker was present to start with and any improvement in Peony's speech would be recorded each day. Key words and situations would be reused. After 2 weeks this strategy would be reviewed to see if Peony had started to copy any of the words or phrases.

Strategy 2
Three new story books using the Sylvannian family stories would be used, both individually and with the whole group. The group would be encouraged to take part in

dramatisations of the stories and Peony would be encouraged to take part, initially in a non-speaking role, but gradually building up her part.

Strategy 3
New songs would be introduced to the group and careful attention would be paid to try to encourage Peony to learn the new words with the other children. The songs would be chosen carefully to introduce elements of humour to try to make them particularly appealing to Peony. Old favourites would be used with instrument sounds replacing key words. Peony would be encouraged to join in with the instruments and everyone would be encouraged to use the words. By working on Peony's likes and strengths, her speech gradually improved.

In the following scenario, critical incident analysis becomes a matter of recording every time a child uses his right hand.

Case Study

Kevin is approaching 18 months, and due to an accident when he was 6 months old, he has restricted use of his right hand. The hand is now healing but he is showing considerable reluctance to use it. He has compensated by using his left hand and has become very adept at this. He is a bright cheerful toddler who, although not speaking in clear words, can make his needs known: by indicating and using various sounds he has learnt that his mother will respond by placing what he wants in front of him.

Before his accident Kevin always sucked his right thumb and would initially reach for objects with his right hand. This could be a sign that his natural hand is the right one. Although being ambidextrous is very useful, he needs to be stimulated to use whichever hand feels most comfortable and natural to him.

Strategies to encourage use of Kevin's right hand:

- *Always place objects to his right*
- *Use large or heavy pieces of equipment so that Kevin uses both hands*
- *Introduce equipment with dials that work in a clockwise direction*
- *Always offer items to Kevin using both hands*
- *Introduce drawing implements*
- *Play at rolling a large ball backwards and forwards.*

A detailed record would be needed to ascertain whether Kevin was using his right more in general and whether the dominance of the right hand was returning.

Conclusion

Observation is an essential tool in early years settings as it enables us to assess individual children, standards within a group, the effectiveness of particular activities or how a piece of equipment is used. However, it is important to be aware of possible shortcomings:

- *Norms of development relate to the progress of an 'average' child and so may not be suitable for use with all children*
- *Norms can give a negative picture of children's achievements – it is better to concentrate on what children can do*
- *Norms allow us to focus in on particular aspects of children's development, but do not give a clear picture of the whole child*
- *Children may not act naturally if they are unused to being watched*
- *We may observe what we expect to see, not what actually happens*
- *We may not be able to take an objective stance when evaluating our observations*
- *Parents may be alarmed by your intention to observe their child – you need to explain sensitively and carefully in order to gain their permission*
- *It is not enough to observe, to be useful observations must be used to inform planning and assess the outcomes of activities.*

6: ASSESSMENT AND RECORDING

Key Points & Introduction

- Utilising observations as the first step towards assessment of the child as a whole
- Assessment as an ongoing process
- The importance of the involvement of other professionals

- Examples of assessment methods
- Planning from assessment – providing the right opportunities for individual development/Evaluating – is the plan working?/Reviewing – what is the next stage?

In the previous chapter we looked at the various methods of observation which are used to build a picture of a whole child and to assess their individual needs. The aim of observation is to gather sufficient information to make the required judgements or *assessments* about the child's stage of development and what activities should be provided to encourage progress. This strategy of observation followed by assessment and recording should be applied to all children in all circumstances, including children with special educational needs.

Initial assessments

What can the child do now?

The method used for an initial assessment identifies the child's own strengths and weaknesses. This has to been done very carefully to ensure that the child really does need special support in one or more areas. Comparison with the child's peers will give valuable, but not conclusive, evidence. Many checklists which assess developmental ages and stages have been produced. One of the hardest decisions to make about children with specific needs is whether that need is sufficient to warrant professional support or not – the dividing line can be very hard to define. In an ideal world every child would have a specially designed educational programme geared to their individual strengths and weaknesses. However, available resources do not provide such a system. It is the function of panels, set up by each Local Education Authority, to decide:

- *Whether a particular child needs support*
- *The level to which the child is supported, bearing in mind any budget restraints and the number of children for whom that budget has to provide.*

The entry profile

One form of initial assessment is the Entry Profile, usually completed when a child starts to attend any type of early years provision. This sheet gives vital information to the setting about the child's level of development.

The completion of such a document would normally be carried out by a parent or carer and discussed with the child's keyworker. The child's introduction to the setting would be governed by the setting's settling in policy.

Table 6.1   A blank entry profile

NAME [ ]   AGE [ ]   DATE [ ]

I like looking at books: ☐ sometimes   ☐ often   ☐ never

my favourite stories are: _____

I like playing with the following toys/activities/people:

at playgroup   at home

_____   _____

_____   _____

_____   _____

I can: ☐ scribble   ☐ draw   ☐ form some letters   ☐ write my name

My imaginative play mostly involves: _____

_____

I like: ☐ singing familiar songs and rhymes ☐ learning new songs and rhymes

☐ climbing on the frame   ☐ playing outside ☐ playing in the home corner

☐ doing puzzles   ☐ making models ☐ painting

playing with   ☐ sand   ☐ water   ☐ clay   ☐ dough

My favourite activity is: _____

I can put on my: ☐ shoes and fasten them   ☐ socks   ☐ clothes and fasten them

I can take off my: ☐ shoes   ☐ socks   ☐ clothes

I like playing mostly: ☐ on my own ☐ with a special friend ☐ with lots of different children

☐ with adults ☐ with siblings

I ask questions about: _____

I can carry out instructions and take messages ☐ sometimes   ☐ often   ☐ not yet

I am happy when _____

I am sad when _____

I am looking forward to _____

I get cross when _____

I get worried about _____

I am frightened by _____

I don't like _____

Best of all I like _____

Case Study

Peter's Entry Profile and development

Name Peter Yobreadth
DOB 18.8.97
Month of Entry September 1999
Address 37 Seriph Avenue, Wentoverton, Stophshire
Telephone 01555 667757
Note if any special circumstance or stage of Code of Practice – *none*
Note if outside agencies involved – *no*
Attendance pattern {if this changes add note} am/(pm) M (T) W (Th) F
Home visit

- Peter is an only child. He had meningitis at the age of 18 months following an ear infection, but made a quick recovery. He likes playing with cars very much, but is quieter than before he was ill. He has become slightly clingy to mum and grandma, who share looking after him – mum works two days a week. His favourite toy is Bert from Sesame Street and he very much likes watching this programme, usually with grandma. His mother thinks his development is normal for his age group and now wants him to attend a nursery two mornings a week, whilst she is at work. This is partly to relieve her mother and particularly to encourage Peter to mix with other children. Peter's parents have chosen this nursery because of its policy of small groups in view of Peter's lack of general socialisation with other children. He has never attended a parent and toddler group and his knowledge of other children is limited to playing with his cousins at weekends. The cousins are two girls, Ruthie and Joanna, who are aged five and seven respectively.
- Peter's parents say he likes to play games – hide and seek in particular – look at books and listen to story tapes.
- The family have a pet cat, Biggles, and a Basset Hound called Freda. Peter is very fond of them both and will often curl up with Freda when he wants a nap.
- Peter's sleep pattern was very good as a baby, but it has been more disturbed since his illness. He often wakes up during the early hours of the morning. He will be comforted by a cuddle and reassurance from either parent, but continually states that he would like to sleep with mummy and daddy, although they have resisted temptation and ensure that Peter remains in his own bed.
- Peter is 'faddy' (his grandma's description) with food and drinks. He

dislikes milk, and prefers juices or water. He is also unwilling to try new foods. He particularly likes cheese, pasta, potatoes and pulses. He is not keen on meat or green vegetables and will not eat fish.

- Peter sucks his thumb a lot. This habit started in hospital and remains a real need for Peter. He prefers his left thumb, but either will do.
- Peter's language was not very clear to me during the home visit, but he has no problem making his needs known to his parents or grandma. His understanding of language seems to be okay. I note that both parents and grandma have excellent diction and talk naturally at a slower place than might be regarded as normal.

Table 6.2   Assessments at 3 years

Ticksheet:
- Recognises:
  - Name   ☐
  - Colours   ☐
  - Belongings [coat etc.]   ☐
- Puts on shoes   ☐
- Toilets alone   ☐
- Sings simple songs from memory   ☐
- Holds pencil, paintbrush and scissors   ☐
- Communicates with other children in constructed sentences   ☐
- Can follow simple instructions   ☐
- Is the child settled in?   ☐

These are detailed comments on Peter's language and literacy made by his keyworker in the October after his first half term:

1. Peter responds to his own name, but sometimes seems to be day-dreaming and takes longer to respond than his peers.
2. He enjoys role play on his own with cars. He becomes a spectator whenever other children join in, or are encouraged to join in. He will play with his keyworker, but loses his interest if keyworker is distracted or called away, and will not return to activity.
3. Peter enjoys using the interest table and was particularly fascinated by the recent table that looked at wheels and had lots of bits and pieces that moved.

4. Peter uses language only when he has to. He responds to direct instructions but can be seen observing the other children and following their lead.

5. Peter will happily point to pictures, but does not say the word back. He will miss about 40% of wrong triggers – if the keyworker uses the wrong word to describe an object Peter will not correct her.

6. Peter enjoys looking at books on his own but shows little interest in following a story in a group situation.

7. No.

8. Peter is still at the scribbling stage, which is acceptable for his age group.

9. No.

10. Peter knows his own name card.

This was summarised to Peter's parents as follows:

Language and Literacy
Peter has enjoyed his first half term and has been very keen to explore his new world. He can recognise his own name and enjoys playing with his keyworker. He enjoys looking at books, but is not ready to sit and listen in group story time yet. We will aim to work at developing his clarity of speech and widen his vocabulary.

Mathematics
Peter enjoys making up patterns and is beginning to show understanding of numbers one to three. He will put pictures into a sequence and can sort by colour, shape and simple definitions.

Personal and Social Development
Peter responds well to his keyworker and plays happily alongside his peers. He can use the toilet by himself and wash and dry his hands.

Creative Development
Peter seems to enjoy drawing, particularly with felt tip pens and we will be encouraging him to spend longer at such activities as appropriate to his age and stage of development. He enjoys watching all that is going on.

Movement
Peter is beginning to enjoy trikes. He has not yet made a definite preference as to which hand to use. He very much likes exploring water and sand.

Knowledge and understanding of the world
Peter is very interested in cars and things that move and will spend lots of time looking and experimenting with construction toys.

Peter's keyworker wrote these notes in preparation for a discussion with the Nursery Manager:

Language and literacy
Peter has difficulty in saying all double consonants and the letter 's'. I have spoken to Grandma on two occasions, but she says she can understand him very well and he is 'chattering away' all the time at home. Mum has now gone back to work full-time, so Grandma is with Peter all the while. When working with Peter, I ensure that he can see my mouth all the time and make sure that I am enunciating correctly. Peter is very reluctant to repeat words, even if they are new words, and we make a game of using them. I have tried including Peter in small group activities when we look at picture cards and talk about the picture, introducing new subjects as appropriate, and when all the children are encouraged to repeat the word back to me. Peter will try occasionally to repeat things, usually without success, following which he will not try again. I have tried getting things wrong on purpose to show that everyone does it and to make light of non-achievement. He will sometimes smile at my efforts but not join in with the laughter that results when I get something very wrong, e.g. 'This is a hat' instead of 'cat'.

I would like to arrange to carry out some specific observations and set up some individual games with Peter over the first two weeks of the Spring term to assess his language capabilities.

Following the meeting with his keyworker, the Nursery Manager wrote to Peter's parents and explained that staff had concerns about his language, and would like to help by investigating this further. Peter's mother said if there were any concerns, she would be prepared to seek outside help from a speech therapist, but felt personally that Peter was just a late developer as far as speech was concerned and that experience with her nieces led her to believe that his speech would develop rapidly after the age of three.

The keyworker carried out a series of four observations during one week — two at each session Peter was attending. One observation involved focussing on his language whilst working with an adult, and another when he was with other children.

The conclusions were:

- Peter follows instructions if they are regular, that is part of the normal regime of the session. He follows the other children when they tidy up, move onto another activity or wash their hands. He will also follow instructions when approached personally and explained one-to-one, at face level, and with slow diction. If an instruction was given over his head as happened on five occasions during the observations, he did not follow them.

- During a recognition game Peter nodded every time he was asked, 'Do you know what this is?' He did not respond verbally to, 'What is this?' He lost interest when asked to repeat the word and began to look round the room and suck his thumb.

- Peter was very reluctant to join in a sounds game using letter sounds: 'Go and find something beginning with (phonic sound). Eventually, he was persuaded to join in with an adult encouraging him to look round and ask questions about particular items. His level of achievement was about 50% when offered direct choice of two objects: 'Let's find something beginning with "t". Shall we choose the teapot or the saucer?'

- It was very difficult to get Peter to join in with making sounds and I did not choose to do this in any great depth because he was becoming agitated with me and the activity. However, overall I would say that his sounds were always a little out, sounding generally lower than the example given and not as prolonged. 'S' or 's' double consonants at the beginning of words caused Peter the most difficulty and other double consonants, 'th', 'chi', 'tr', 'cr' in particular were not recognisable.

- The Nursery manager wrote again to Peter's parents and asked if both or either of them could come into the Nursery to discuss Peter's speech with both her and the keyworker. Peter's mother wrote back that she was very busy at the present time, but that her mother had agreed to keep the appointment. Grandma was very reluctant to see that Peter was not achieving. She felt that he was very young, that speech would develop naturally with age and that to keep testing him was unfair and unsettling. She agreed to feedback the keyworker's findings to Peter's parents.

- Peter's parents arranged for him to see a speech therapist privately and she produced a report which suggested strategies to work with Peter. However, Peter's parents are also concerned about Peter being put under pressure and have requested a change of keyworker.

Following completion of an entry profile at the start of nursery education, the following checklists can be useful.

Table 6.3   Assessment at 4 years

Mathematics

Tick sheet:

- Can s/he count? How many?   ☐   _____
- Can s/he match numbers to items?   ☐
- Does s/he join in number rhymes?   ☐
- What shapes does s/he know?   ☐
    - Triangle?   ☐
    - Square?   ☐
    - Rectangle?   ☐
    - Circle?   ☐
- Can she/he put things in order?
    - Tallest, shortest?   ☐
    - Biggest, smallest?   ☐
    - Long, short?   ☐
    - In front of, behind?   ☐

Creative

- Does the child know primary colours?   ☐
  Does the child know other colours, e.g. black, white, gold, silver, purple?   ☐
- Can the child: ☐
    - Match by colour, shape and size?   ☐
    - Do a simple jigsaw?   ☐
    - Pick the odd one out?   ☐
    - Draw a person with arms, legs, facial details?   ☐
    - Draw a house?   ☐
    - Identify different textures, e.g. rough and smooth?   ☐

Knowledge and understanding of the world

- Does the child know:
    - Their address?   ☐
    - Their phone number?   ☐
    - The names of their brothers, sisters?   ☐
    - How old they are?   ☐
    - Their grandparents?   ☐

Table 6.3 Assessment at 4 years (cont'd)

- Transport:
  - Does the child know how they got to playgroup today, e.g. walking, car, bus, train? ☐
- Pets and animals:
  - Can the child name their pet? ☐
  - Does she know about mother and baby animals? ☐
  - Can s/he name farm animals? ☐
  - Does s/he know about trees and plants? ☐
- Weather:
  - Can the child describe the weather today, e.g. hot, cold, wet, dry? ☐
- Clothes:
  - Can the child describe what s/he is wearing today? ☐

- Can the child make:
  - Facial expressions? ☐
  - Body prints? ☐
  - Hand prints? ☐
  - Foot prints? ☐

Physical Development

	Poor	Satisfactory	Good	Comments
● Climbing frame	☐	☐	☐	
● Trampoline	☐	☐	☐	
● Tunnels	☐	☐	☐	
● Catching	☐	☐	☐	
● Throwing	☐	☐	☐	
● Music and movement	☐	☐	☐	
● Instrument playing	☐	☐	☐	
● Hoops (rolling)	☐	☐	☐	
● Bikes and scooters	☐	☐	☐	
● Hopping on one leg	☐	☐	☐	
● Jumping	☐	☐	☐	
● Skipping	☐	☐	☐	
● Running	☐	☐	☐	
● Pushing and pulling	☐	☐	☐	
● Sand	☐	☐	☐	
● Dough (imaginative play)	☐	☐	☐	
● Clay	☐	☐	☐	
● Scissors	☐	☐	☐	

Table 6.3 Assessment at 4 years (cont'd)

	Poor	Satisfactory	Good	Comments
• Pencil control	☐	☐	☐	
• Threads beads or pegs	☐	☐	☐	

Personal and Social
- Recognises name on peg ☐
- Takes coat off and hangs on peg ☐
- Puts on coat, does up buttons ☐
- Toilets alone ☐
- Washes hands ☐
- Relates to others ☐
- Shares with others ☐
- Knows right from wrong ☐
- Understands instructions ☐
- Takes turns in a group ☐
- Is helpful and kind ☐
- Says please and thank you ☐
- Is polite ☐
- Shows self confidence ☐

Language and Literacy
- Understands what is said ☐
- Follows simple instructions ☐
- Takes a message ☐
- Understands books go from left to right ☐
- Follows text ☐
- Can relate stories to adults ☐
- Can tell a simple story using pictures ☐
- Knows a number of nursery rhymes, songs and poems ☐
- Recognises own name ☐
- Can write some or all of name ☐
- Recognises some letters ☐
- Can name well-known objects when labelled ☐
- Recognises rhymes and rhyming sounds, e.g. cat, mat, sat ☐
- Answers questions with: ☐
  - A gesture ☐
  - One word ☐
  - A sentence ☐
- Can carry on a simple conversation ☐

Figure 6.1
Rocket record of
achievement

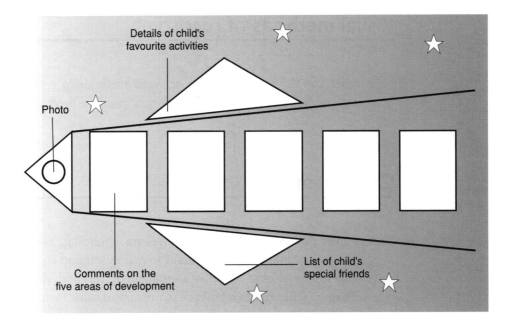

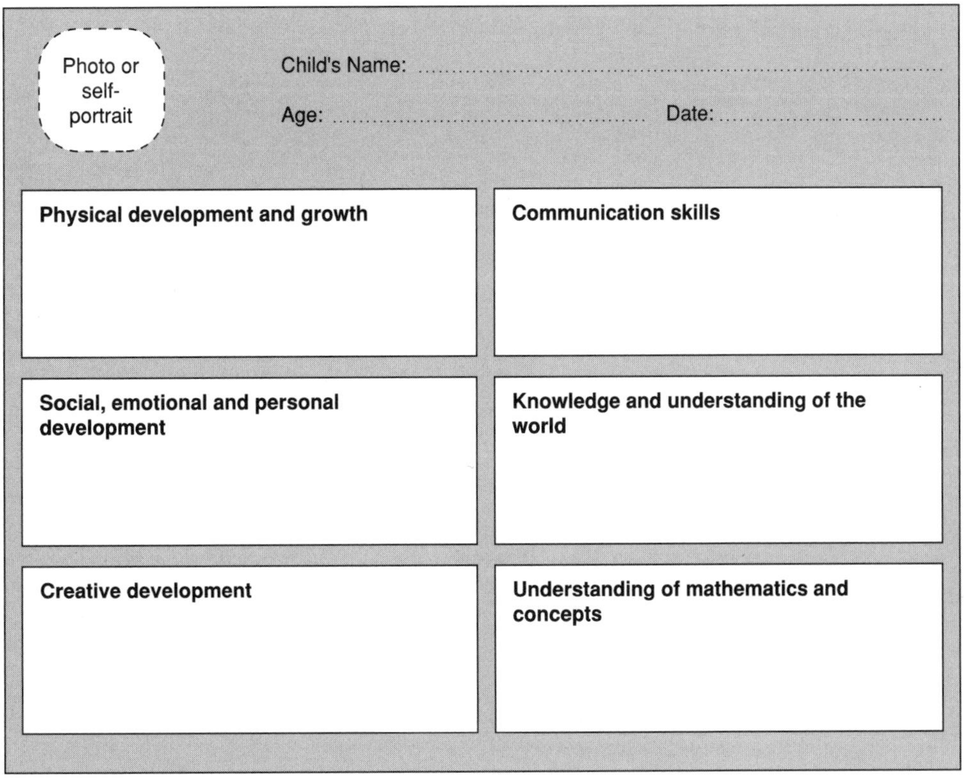

Details of child's
favourite activities

Photo

Comments on the
five areas of development

List of child's
special friends

Figure 6.2
**Photo or self-
portrait**

Photo or
self-
portrait

Child's Name: ....

Age: .... Date: ....

Physical development and growth

Communication skills

**Social, emotional and personal
development**

**Knowledge and understanding of the
world**

Creative development

**Understanding of mathematics and
concepts**

Visual methods of recording

Figures 6.1 and 6.2 show examples of visual methods of recording assessment, to which the children can contribute. This format could be used as both 'initial' and also ongoing.

Conclusion

This chapter provides a selection of forms for observing, assessing and recording. When observing children it is important to make clear and accurate recordings. This will enable you to make an objective assessment of the child. Remember that you and your colleagues will need to refer back to previous records to assess progress.

7: COLLABORATION WITH OTHER PROFESSIONALS

Key Points & Introduction

- Who are the professionals that early years workers can expect to collaborate with?
- How and where do we find these professionals when we need them?
- What will they do to help the child?

- How can I support the work that the professional and the child do together?
- What contact will the parents or carer have with the professional?
- How will we all share information?

There is a variety of professionals whose job it is to support children with special educational needs, their parents and their early years workers. In order to care effectively for children it is important to be aware of the full range of services and to be able to work alongside others. The value of teamwork and interagency cooperation cannot be overestimated. It is always helpful to share responsibility and coordinate a response when action for a child is required. We need to take the opportunity to meet and exchange information on current practice with other early years professionals on a regular basis. This will benefit our working relationships and strengthen the support systems available to parents and children. Initial contact with the appropriate professional is made easier if you are aware of their responsibilities and role in the system and can put a face to a name.

Emotions of loneliness, fear, worry and frustration are common feelings for adults as well as children involved in the collaboration. Security can be found in the *sharing* of information with others. A moral dilemma may arise as we proceed in the collaboration, often sharing and receiving confidential information from other professionals and parents. It is important to maintain an objective and professional approach in potentially difficult situations. Remember to work always with the best interests of the child in mind.

The professionals

Early years workers may come across a whole range of people through their work with children with special educational needs:

Figure 7.1
Where do we find
these professionals?

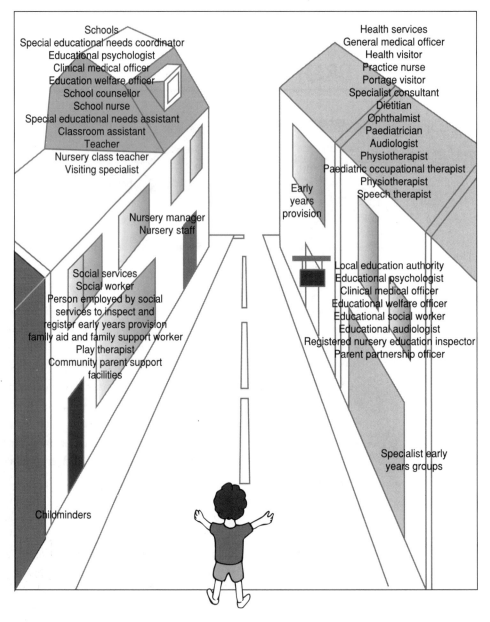

Schools
Special educational needs coordinator
Educational psychologist
Clinical medical officer
Education welfare officer
School counsellor
School nurse
Special educational needs assistant
Classroom assistant
Teacher
Nursery class teacher
Visiting specialist

Health services
General medical officer
Health visitor
Practice nurse
Portage visitor
Specialist consultant
Dietitian
Ophthalmist
Paediatrician
Audiologist
Physiotherapist
Paediatric occupational therapist
Physiotherapist
Speech therapist

Early
years
provision

Nursery manager
Nursery staff

Social services
Social worker
Person employed by social
services to inspect and
register early years provision
family aid and family support worker
Play therapist
Community parent support
facilities

Local education authority
Educational psychologist
Clinical medical officer
Educational welfare officer
Educational social worker
Educational audiologist
Registered nursery education inspector
Parent partnership officer

Specialist early
years groups

Childminders

Educational audiologist
Nursery nurse
Paediatric occupational therapist
Physiotherapist
Playgroup or Preschool supervisor
Preschool manager
Senior medical technical officer

Special educational needs coordinator
Special needs assistant
Specialist educational psychologist
Speech and language therapist
Voluntary Portage worker.

In order to help us discover more about the roles and responsibilities of these professionals we will now look at five short descriptions and weekly diaries submitted by the professionals themselves.

The educational audiologist

I am an educational audiologist and I have been working with children who have special educational needs for 13 years. I trained as a teacher of English and drama and also have training in audiology (the science of hearing). I work part-time, about 10 to 14 hours each week, and am directly involved with 93 children. As part of a team, I work with other agencies such as Health Authorities, Creative and Performing Arts organisations and Services for the Learning Impaired. I enjoy working with the children and showing visitors around the school, but the report writing and administration requirements of my work are less enjoyable.

Figure 7.2
An educational
audiologist at work
with a child

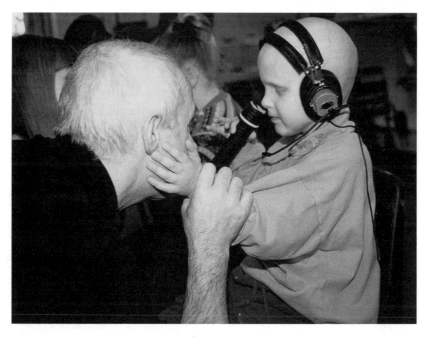

A typical week

Monday:

  8.45–9.15 am Briefing with audiology technician

  9.15–9.45 Music with primary 1

  9.45–10.15 Music with primary 2

10.15–10.50 Music with primary 3

11.00–11.30 Music with multi-sensory primary

11.30–12.00 pm Music with multi-sensory senior

  1.00–1.30 Music with extended education (+ 19 years)

  1.30–3.00 Music with secondary 3 and 4

  3.00–5.00 Administration

Tuesday:

  8.45–9.15 am Briefing with audiology technician

  9.30–12.00 pm Clinic-based audiological assessment

12.00–12.45 Report writing

  1.15–2.30 Audiological assessment

  2.30–5.00 INSET planning and assessment preparation

Wednesday:

  8.45–9.15 am Briefing with audiology technician

  9.15–12.00 pm Audiological assessment

12.00–12.45 Report writing

  1.30–2.30 Audiological assessment

  2.30–5.00 Administration and curriculum meetings

Thursday:

  8.45–9.15 am Briefing with audiology technician   or

  9.30–10.00 Informal class-based hearing assessment   All day

10.00–12.00 pm Showing visitors around the school   external

12.00–12.45 Administration   assessment

  1.30–3.00 Class-based hearing assessment

  3.00–5.00 Planning and debrief with educational psychologist

Friday:

  8.45–9.15 am Briefing with audiology technician   or

  9.15–11.00 Assessment team meeting   Delivery of

11.00–12.45 pm Report writing   INSET,

  1.30–2.30 Department meeting   internal or

  2.30–5.00 Research project with educational psychologist   external

The nursery nurse

I am a qualified nursery nurse working in a purpose-built playcentre for children with special needs. The centre is a registered charity and we provide weekday care throughout the year for approximately 250 children aged 1 month to 5 years. I have been involved with children who have special educational needs for 2 years and am employed full-time for 35 hours each week.

At present I work with 29 children during the morning session and 32 in the afternoon session. Other professionals are involved in the centre and I work with speech therapists, physiotherapists and occupational therapists. We use a variety of teaching methods and resources depending upon the needs of the children: Signalong and Derbyshire language, physiotherapy programmes and exercises for standing and sitting using standing frames, chairs and sensory stimulation equipment. My training has included first aid, a preliminary instructors' qualification in swimming, food hygiene and a variety of other staff training opportunities. I enjoy playing and interacting with the children. The most difficult part of my work is coming to terms with some of the children's conditions. Some children get progressively worse. Occasionally, children die.

A typical week
Monday to **Thursday**
am
The morning sessions are attended by 29 children with a variety of special needs and conditions, for example cerebral palsy, West syndrome, Down's syndrome and visual and hearing impairments. We offer a variety of activities to suit the differing levels of ability and development.
9.15 am Children arrive with parents or in centre mini buses – I support the children during freeplay in the main playroom
10.30 Drinks time.
11.00 Nappy change time.
11.15 I work in the sensory room using lights and soft play equipment.
11.30 Group singing time.
11.45 Home time.

pm
The afternoon sessions are attended by 32 children. The majority attend for social reasons, for example behavioural problems, speech and language delay or housing environments resulting in play restrictions.
1.00 pm Children arrive with parents or in centre mini buses – I support the children during freeplay in the main playroom
1.20 Potty training and nappy change

1.45–2.15 Group activities such as sensory song, cookery, art, sand and water play, music and movement, garden play or a neighbourhood walk.

2.30 Drinks time

2.45 Singing

3.00 Home time

On Friday afternoons the centre is closed. Staff meet to plan and prepare for the following week. We also change wall displays and clean and check materials and equipment.

The paediatric occupational therapist

I am a paediatric occupational therapist and I have been working with children with special educational needs for 2 years. I have a BSc in Occupational Therapy and have attended various courses. I am employed by a school for the deaf for about 7 hours each week and I also work in community provisions for about 30 hours each week. Other professionals and agencies I work with are equipment manufacturers, wheelchair clinics and the Social Services department. I am part of a therapy team. At present I am working with seven children using therapeutic techniques in daily life situations such as toileting. My role is to encourage the children to fulfil their functional potential using hands-on therapeutic intervention and adaptations to their environment.

A typical week

Monday

Working in the community all day. Special and mainstream schools, assessment centres and home visits.

Tuesday

Working in the community during the morning and at a special school in the afternoon.

Wednesday

As Tuesday.

Thursday

Working with further education students in the morning and extension education students in the afternoon. Assessment of functional seating and equipment needs when possible.

Friday

Assessments at the local hospital in the morning. Community and administration work in the afternoon.

Figure 7.3
A paediatric
occupational
therapist in a session
with a child

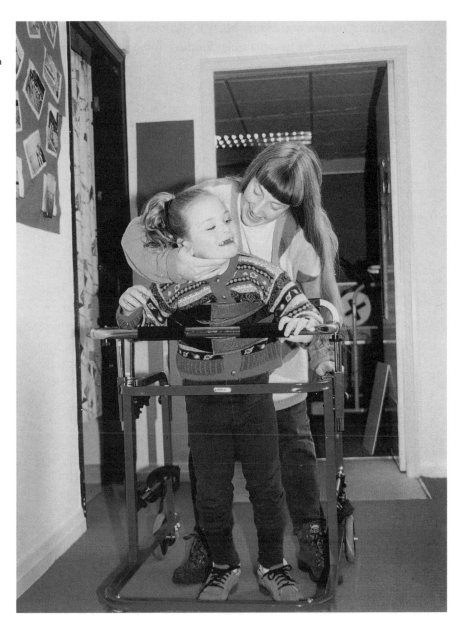

The physiotherapist

I am a physiotherapist and have been working with children with special educational needs for 9 years. I work approximately 36 hours each week and am involved with a total of 80 children. As part of a team, I am involved with other professionals such as consultants, occupational therapists and community therapists. I have completed training on physiotherapy, MOVE, orthotics and orthopaedics. The most difficult part of my work is obtaining funding for equipment, but I enjoy the hands-on management of students.

A typical week

Monday
9.00–11.00 am I support in the multi-sensory unit
11.00–12.00 pm MOVE
12.00–1.00 Administration, telephone calls and report writing
1.00–2.00 Walk and gym
2.00–3.00 PE with CP children
3.00 I support in residential units

Tuesday
9.00–11.00 am I support in the multi-sensory unit
11.00–12.00 pm Administration work
1.00–3.00 MOVE
3.00 I support in the residential units

Wednesday
am Administration work
1.00–2.00 pm MOVE
2.00 Staff training

Thursday
9.00–11.00 am I support in the multi-sensory unit
11.00–12.00 MOVE
1.00–2.00 PE
2.00–3.00 Administration work

Friday
am Orthotic clinic and departmental meetings
pm Contact with parents by telephone and home books

The playgroup supervisor

I am a playgroup supervisor and have worked with children with special needs for 14 years. My qualification is a Diploma in Playgroup Practice and I have also attended a variety of training days to inform me about special educational needs. I work 9 hours each week with a total of 32 children using 'see and say' signing and special pieces of equipment such as standing frames. I am part of a team and work with other professionals and agencies. These may include a speech therapist, physiotherapist, health visitors and doctors. The children have a wide range of needs such as language and communication disorders, hearing impairment and delayed development. I enjoy supervising the sessions and working with the children. The most difficult part of my work is helping parents to come to terms with their child's special need and dealing with the endless paperwork.

A typical week
Monday
Closed

Tuesday to Friday
8.45 am Arrive to set up the hall
9.45 Welcome children as they arrive and speak to parents
Until 10.45 I organise and help the children with their individual needs through play. Once a week during the morning session, some children receive speech therapy either individually or in small groups. A physiotherapist also works with some of the children once a week.
10.45 I reorganise the hall and change the activities and equipment while the children have their refreshments
11.30 Staff and children clear away the equipment and sit in a circle for singing time
12.00 pm Parents arrive to collect the children

The preschool supervisor

I am a preschool supervisor. In April, 1986 I attended a toddler group with my son and in the same year I had started to help out. This progressed until July 1991, when I took over the running of the group. I had helped out at various playgroups as a volunteer helper between 1986 and 1992, one of which was an opportunity group. The opportunity group encourages children with disabilities or learning difficulties to play alongside other children. For one term I held a post as a temporary assistant. Since September 1993, I have been the principal of a preschool group. At this group we encourage all children to attend whether they have special needs or not. I have had a variety of experience with children with special needs including asthma, autism, partial sight, hearing impairment, speech difficulties, hyperactivity, emotional and social problems and having English as a second language. One child had a brain tumour which resulted in the left side of his body not being developed. I have a variety of qualifications which include the Diploma in Playgroup Practice, NVQ Level 3 in Childcare and Education and I am an NVQ assessor. Courses I have attended include Child Protection, First Aid, National Curriculum for Early Years and Special Needs training, including a Portage seminar. I enjoy being with the children, but finding the funding for extra staff is the most difficult part of my work. All in all, I have worked for 12 years with children. At present I work for 10 hours a week with 44 children, 16 of whom have special educational needs. The most rewarding part of my work is seeing the children progress.

The preschool manager

A typical week

Monday

I arrive at 8.00 am. The milk order is wrong again so I call the dairy. I open the mail and check the answering machine. The desk diary shows a new child starts today, we have two birthdays to celebrate and the librarian will visit to read stories to the children. I find the floorplan for today's programme of activities, the timetable and the staff rota and place them all on the desk. I pin a reminder on the parents' information board about Sports Day arrangements and a notification of a head lice outbreak.

Staff arrive at 8.30. We have a coffee and discuss the paperwork on the desk and any other business such as observations of children. The playroom is set out, kitchen preparations are made for snacktime. I find the register and the paperwork required for the new child.

9.00 We open the door and the noise level rises. Children store their personal belongings, find their name card to give me and I mark the register. Parents and carers are talking to their children's keyworkers and information is recorded in the desk diary, for example if a child is being collected by a different adult. The new child arrives and I introduce parent and child to the chosen keyworker and group after checking personal details with parent. The child's other parent has recently died and I have made several home visits to discuss the child and family's needs. We have agreed a settling in process. In one corner a volunteer parent is running the home book scheme as folders are returned after the weekend and children comment on their chosen book.

9.15 The door is locked as we gather together for newstime, to call the register and talk about the programme for today. Keyworkers sit with their children in groups of four or five and support children with special needs to ensure they are fully involved, especially at newstime and when we acknowledge the two birthdays.

9.30 The group activities are taking place. The weekly theme is senses so each keyworker has planned activities for their group. Some children go out onto the adjoining field to explore and some stay indoors to make scented playdough or play a game.

10.30 Everyone is ready for snacktime and as we are using our sense of smell today, the keyworkers encourage the learning to continue as the children wash their hands with fruit shaped and scented soaps and eat and drink fruity concoctions.

11.00 The librarian rings the door bell.

11.45 Time for ring games and a few songs. Then coats on and time for home. I check the desk diary for parents' instructions. The register is called again and the door is opened for parents to collect the children at 12.00 pm. Staff clear away resources and write up any keyworker records. I eat my packed lunch and prepare for the afternoon session.

12.30 Staff changeover and preparations for afternoon session start with short staff meeting over coffee.

1.00 Ready to open the door again. One staff member is late and I have to take over her group. The staff member arrives one hour late because of car trouble. The planned programme continues until 4.00, then silence. Everyone helps to clean up and we discuss the day's events.

Tuesday

Arrive at 8.00 am to discover two broken windows. Telephone police to report and find insurance policy details. Telephone window repair company to come and board them up. Clean up glass. Staff arrive. Cut finger on piece of glass I have overlooked. Enter details into accident book. Health visitor telephones to arrange a visit to discuss the new child who started yesterday. Letter from child development centre contains activity ideas from paediatric occupational therapist for child who has English as an additional language, poor fine motor skills and short attention span. I pass this onto the child's keyworker after we have discussed the exercises and any resources which would be needed. Usual supervision of morning and afternoon sessions.

Wednesday

Usual supervision of morning and afternoon sessions. Health visitor agreed to meet me before the new child arrived at 9.00 am. Discussed parent and child's responses to first day and looked at keyworker's file. As there are no apparent problems, the health visitor decided to telephone parent and visit child at home.

Thursday

Usual supervision of morning session until 12.00 pm. 1.00–2.30 An afternoon session for parents, carers and toddlers to socialise and share experiences.

6.30 Staff meeting. We have monthly meetings to discuss and look at keyworkers' files, including individual education plans and specialists' reports. Curriculum planning meetings are held every half term and include staff suggestions for new equipment and resources to meet the children's needs. We arrange keyworker and group visits with a card and present for a child in hospital for a minor operation. I have informed the child's parents about the intended visit and they have given written permission.

Friday

Usual morning and afternoon sessions until 4.00 pm. 4.00–5.00 Administration work. I write out open day invitations for the session during half term week when children have play opportunities while parents and carers talk to staff and look at keyworker's files. I display the children's work, including large models and collages that all the children have contributed to.

The senior medical technical officer

I am a senior medical technical officer and I have been involved with children with special needs for 15 years. At present, I am employed 4 days each week for 28 hours in a large school working with approximately 87 children. I work with an educational audiologist, local hospital hearing aid department and audiology clinics throughout the United Kingdom.

A typical week
Monday

am Approximately 16 one-to-one hearing tests with and without hearing aids for annual review reports

pm Administration work, writing reports, getting hearing aids ready to go for repair and hearing aid moulds ready for manufacture

Figure 7.4
Children having their
hearing tested

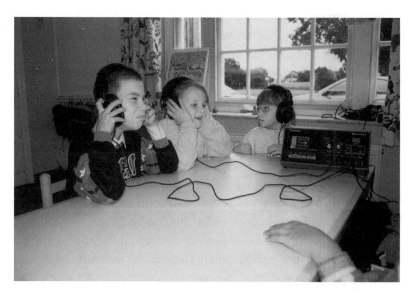

Tuesday

am One-to-one assessments working with educational audiologist
pm Visit local hospital hearing aid department for supplies (the number of these visits each week depends on the amount of equipment for repair and manufacture)

Thursday

I go into classrooms for routine hearing and maintenance work. I work with 4 to 8 children to check their ears and to take away hearing aids for electronic testing. Thursday is assessment day for children referred for advice and placement.

Friday

am One-to-one assessments and routine hearing and maintenance work, listening skills work and work with a variety of listening aids if time allows
pm Administration work in office, training given or received in response to demand

The special educational needs coordinator

Almost all schools have a special educational needs coordinator or SENCO. The responsibility for managing the school's SEN provision is often shared between the SENCO and members of the Senior Management Team. The SENCO is responsible for:

- *The day-to-day operation of the school's SEN policy*
- *Advising class teachers on meeting a range of needs*
- *Coordinating the staged approach to school-based assessment*
- *Maintaining effective record keeping, such as the SEN register, staged assessment targets, medical information and individual education plans (IEPs)*
- *Ensuring the full involvement of parents in decision-making about pupils with SEN*
- *Liaising with external agencies such as Social Services, medical and voluntary organisations*
- *Organising annual reviews, ensuring reports are circulated to all relevant parties and notes on the review are submitted to Local Education Authority.*

The special needs assistant

I am a special needs assistant and a qualified nursery nurse. I have worked in a nursery class for 6 years and during the last year I have been involved with children who have visual impairment. I am employed for about 12 hours each week. My role is to encourage and support the children. My duties include the adaptation of worksheets, writing individual education plans, keeping weekly records, attending staff meetings, working with small groups of children and also one-to-one when other children are copying from the blackboard, for example. I work with other professionals such as the school staff, the special educational needs coordinator and the staff of the special needs centre. I have daily contact with the parents. I am a valued member of the team and if I need advice or support I can approach the special needs centre staff.

A typical week

Monday

I help to collect dinner money. Then I sit with a group of children and listen to the class teacher explain the programme for the day. I sit with a group of seven children, including a child with visual impairment to help write their news. I help with spellings and maths work with the same group.

Tuesday

I work with a teacher from the special needs centre and a group of seven children to improve their sight vocabulary. We prepare sight vocabulary folders for the following

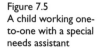
Figure 7.5
A child working one-to-one with a special needs assistant

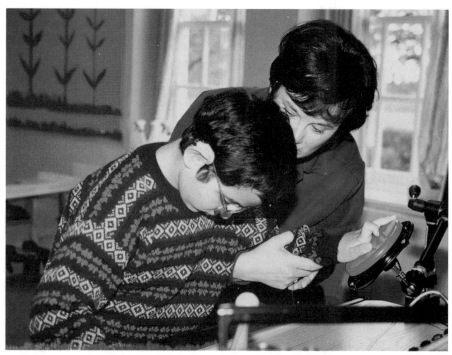

week. I listen to readers. Then I do a science investigation with a group which is working on the topic, capacity.

Wednesday
We have a reading workshop. Parents attend and take small groups of children to read a book, discuss and than complete follow up worksheets. I listen to readers. I encourage and support a child with special needs during a PE lesson.

Thursday
I run an English and maths support group, attend assembly and silent reading. I also help with topic work.

Friday
Again we do English and maths work. I attend assembly, prepare resources and manage activities for art, craft and cookery.

The educational psychologist

I am a specialist educational psychologist. I have worked with children with special educational needs for more than 20 years. My qualifications are an Honours Degree in Psychology, Postgraduate qualification and training in education, attendance at courses over many years on special needs, deafness, communication, assessments and behaviours. I work directly and indirectly with the whole school population of about 95 children who are aged from 4 years to 25 years. The most difficult part of my work is the organising and compiling of complex reports, child protection investigations and the support of staff who are managing challenging behaviours. I enjoy working with colleagues, sharing the children's successes with parents and attending annual reviews. Other professionals I work with include a psychiatrist, a behaviour management coordinator, an audiologist, a physiotherapist, an occupational therapist, a general language therapist and others in relation to assessments and annual reviews.

A typical week
Monday
Annual reviews all day. Chair meetings and write review reports. Preparation for reviews, reading files and consulting with school staff. Discussion with local authority representatives, hearing impaired service, social workers, education office and parents.

Tuesday
am Class visits for observations and discussion with teachers. Preparing reports for

transitional reviews. Administration including returning telephone calls and following up requests for assessments and visits.

pm Prepare information for psychological reports. Meeting with colleagues, audiologist, teacher and head of department.

Wednesday

am External visit to school in adjoining authority to observe a child who has been referred for assessment. Discussion with head and class teacher.

pm Meeting with parents and teacher of a school child to discuss behaviour management and decide action.

Thursday

Multidisciplinary assessment with audiologist, physiotherapist and occupational therapist to include period of observation and assessment of a child, discussion with parents and feedback of information obtained that day. After school visit to a residential unit to observe and discuss a student.

Friday

am Administration. Preparation and collection of interdisciplinary assessment reports. Researching files in preparation for next week's reviews and meetings.

pm Interim review for student in transition. Chair and write report of meeting.

The following form is an example of the type of information I require to make an assessment of a child who has been referred to me.

Pupil's Name:

DOB:

Age:

SEN Stage:

School:

Consultation Between:

For example class teacher, head teacher.

Date:

Details From Previous Consultation:

Nature of Current Involvement:

For example initial information sharing, assessment of situation or needs, review and evaluation.

Consultation Objectives:
For example, Individual Education Plan, targets for pupil, intervention strategies.

Method:
For example, shared discussion, observation, involvement with child, individually, in group or in class.

Summary:
For example, aggression towards staff and peers.

Agreed Further Action Checklist:
For example, contact behaviour management team for advice.

Aims/Targets:
For example, to decrease incidents of aggression, pinching and biting.

Strategies/Action:
For example, to devise a behaviour programme, adult to emphasise general class rules, praise positive behaviour, anticipate problem trigger especially groupwork.

Personnel Involved in Above:
For example, parents, class teacher.

Total Consultation Time:

Further Consultation: Yes/No

The speech and language therapist

I am a speech and language therapist with approximately 10 years experience. I graduated from university with a B. Med. Sci (Speech) Hons. which was a 4 year speech pathology undergraduate degree course. I have been employed for the past 6 years by the Healthcare National Health Service Trust, working with preschool and school children with moderate and severe learning difficulties. I work with preschool children with physical difficulties and also children with feeding difficulties. The ages of the children on my caseload range from 3 weeks to 19 years.

I work in a variety of settings including the children's own homes, special schools and the local child development centre. Where I see the children depends on a variety of factors including their age and their communication difficulty. As the majority of the children on my caseload are seen by several different professionals regular liaison is essential and, when appropriate, I see children jointly with others such as the child's Portage worker, the dietitian, the physiotherapist or the occupational therapist. Parental involvement is encouraged and is usually a key factor in the success of any intervention. Parents are provided with regular written reports on their child's progress which, with their consent, are also copied to all professionals known to be involved with their child. For the children who receive their speech and language therapy input at school, the parents are always informed of the appointment and are invited either to attend or to contact me to discuss their child's difficulties.

A typical week
Monday
Working at school assessing, observing and making formal assessments where possible. I have discussions with the class teacher and parents to go over my findings and to plan aims. I demonstrate activities to work towards achieving the aims we have agreed. I also write down programmes explaining the activities. I write reports on children I have seen that day and update my case notes. Liaison with school staff is important.

Tuesday
Today, I have home visits and joint assessments with less experienced speech and language therapists providing support for them. I attend the child development centre for regular therapy sessions with children with complex needs.

Wednesday
As Monday.

Thursday
am as Tuesday.
pm Administration work and meetings.

Friday
am Child development centre as Tuesday.
pm Attend some appointments, sometimes made jointly with Portage workers.
   The following is an extract from one of my reports.

Chronological age: 5 years 2 months   *Name of G.P.*: Dr Clark
Comments on Assessment:
This child has had two visits for assessment. The child presented as chatty and
confident, and was enthusiastic throughout the assessment. The formal assessments
were administered and their findings are as follows below.

Reynell Development Language Scale (Comprehension):
Age equivalent: 5 years 6 months to 5 years 8 months
Results show an improvement on last test approximately 11 months ago which
placed child a year below the chronological age.

Renfrew Action Picture Test:
Information score: 33 (27–33 is within normal limits)
Grammar Score: 18 (19–26 is within normal limits)
Child's grammar is a little immature. Child also made semantic errors for example,
'The cat bounced on the fence' (instead of jumped).

The Portage worker

I am a voluntary Portage worker and have worked with children with special
educational needs for the last 15 months. I have been involved with young children
for many years, beginning by setting up a playgroup. After giving up a full-time
professional post, I trained in early years work. I was a support worker for a voluntary
organisation, visiting local playgroups, nurseries and parent and toddler groups.
Following this, I was employed by Social Services as an assistant Under 8's
Advisor, again visiting and supporting groups, but with the added responsibility of
registering and inspecting early years provision and childminders.

Recently, I received 4 days training in Portage and am now involved with a child
for about 2 hours per week. Every 2 weeks I attend a team meeting of voluntary
Portage workers, sometimes with other professionals such as speech therapists, who
advise and support us. I work with the child's family using resources supplied by the
family or myself.

I enjoy identifying the developmental areas requiring attention but finding activities
that address these needs is difficult. Portage is a scheme for teaching preschool
children with special needs new and useful skills in their own home and in a partnership
with their parents. Portage has developed in this country, after being introduced

from America in 1976. There are now approximately 150 registered Portage Services operating in the United Kingdom.

Examples of good practice

Examples of good practice of inclusive education are provided by the special needs assistant who explains special facilities, organisation of special needs provision and classroom strategies provided by her school.

'There is wheelchair access to all parts of the school and a wide range of resources available to support the learning of children with SEN. Specialist teachers work one-to-one with children with special needs, such as hearing or sight impairment. Other professionals who work with the children are educational psychologists who help with assessments and speech and language therapists who advise on provision for the children. Support services include an occupational therapist, the Educational Welfare Service, Social Services Child Guidance Unit and School Health department.

We provide help in the classroom using flexible grouping which allows children of similar abilities to work together. We develop close links between home and school by encouraging parents to be involved with their children's learning. They are often invited to help with classroom activities and in home reading and writing schemes. Parents are included in the volunteer reading scheme and regularly hear children read, spend time talking with them or using the computer in one-to-one situations. Extension exercises are provided for the children who complete their work quickly. This includes opportunities to read stories to the nursery class children and workshops for maths, writing and spelling.

The number of children with special educational needs aged 4 to 6 years attending the school at present and their stages of assessment are as follows:

- *37 children at Stage 1*
- *No children at Stage 2*
- *59 children at Stage 3*
- *1 child at Stage 4*
- *1 child at Stage 5.*'

Sharing information

A successful exchange of information will bring together several disciplines to share ideas and learn from each other. Formal and informal training opportunities for staff, parents and volunteers with specialists promotes understanding and extends communication skills. The more we are informed the more we can support and help the child. To be able to effectively interact and work with other professionals we must have knowledge of the areas of expertise offered by them.

Chapters 5 and 6 illustrate the importance of monitoring children's development through assessment, recording and reporting. The process provides valuable information to pass onto other professionals, as well as being useful for staff to plan curriculum activities and to evaluate the effectiveness of resources. When supplemented with parents' observations from home, these insights can lead a team of professionals to a better understanding of the needs of the child and family. Exchange of information is especially important during any stage of transition, for example when a child returns to the nursery after a long period of absence or changes nursery venues.

Accessing services

There are barriers which can prevent or delay access to services. This can be frustrating and will require persistance.

Limits on finance can prove a barrier to collaboration. Many families will not be able to afford to pay for specialist help. They will require assistance from you to access the services that they are entitled to. Funded access to professionals can only be accomplished by persistence and you should attempt to provide continuity of progress for the child. Parents are usually at the forefront of the drive to obtain help for their child and they often get frustrated at the slowness of the system. It is part of your role to support parents during the wait and to push for action on their behalf.

The voluntary sector provides many support and help groups for children and their families. You should be aware of groups in your area so that you can advise parents accordingly. *Opportunity groups* are one of many services providing help and support for families experiencing frustration as they try to access provision in their local area. There are lots of parent support groups that meet formally and informally, using a variety of accommodation and funded by grants or fundraising events. They provide a valuable service and an oasis for parents and children who need to share experiences with others who understand and to have fun together in a relaxed and caring environment. This personal account from a parent of a child with special needs highlights the value of these voluntary groups.

'My name is Helen and I am the mother of two children, one of whom has special needs. The first support I encountered was from the supervisor of the opportunity group my son and I attended. She was very supportive, always willing to listen and could always tell when I was feeling worried or low. This usually happened when my son was due to be admitted to hospital for an operation. The supervisor supported both the adults and the children who attended the group.

After she left the group I felt very alone and received little or no support from the group when my son had his second kidney operation. I told myself that it was only a minor operation and other children had more serious ones. But I had no relatives nearby to help or give me a break.

Generally on the medical side everything has been good, brilliant even. I have had good support from professionals such as a renal consultant, ophthalmologist, dentist, orthodontist, psychologist, dietitian, physiotherapist, orthopedic surgeon, health visitor, social worker and educational therapist. Mostly the contact was at hospitals such as Great Ormond Street or the Royal Alexander Children's hospital. My child has asthma, growth hormone deficiency and displayed behavioural problems believed to be influenced by his hospital treatment and medical problems. Initially, I did not know where to get help and it was very difficult. Information should be easy to get hold of and there was no one to tell me whom I should go to get help. I got help eventually when the under eights adviser walked into the opportunity group as I was talking to the nurse and I just broke down.

I wish the professionals had listened to what I was saying in the early days. Maybe my son's behaviour and social skills wouldn't have got so bad. Professionals should listen and realised that we are not stupid people who are over-reacting. All we want is the best for our children. The professionals should know that, just because a child doesn't fall into a category in the text book, it doesn't mean nothing is wrong. Parents and carers should not have to fight for what their child needs. Money should not determine whether our children get the support and treatment they need. Information and help should be freely available. Life is stressful enough having a special needs child. If more help is available at the beginning, money would be saved in the long term.'

Children have lots of different needs and have contact with a large number of professionals. These cases highlight the need for effective exchange of information between all parties. This helps to ensure that the child receives appropriate provision, that everybody works with the same aims in mind and that there is the minimum delay. For example, updating records after a child's period of absence from educational provision – perhaps because of a stay in hospital – must be done quickly to ensure appropriate after care is offered.

Conclusion

The list of professionals covered in this chapter is by no means comprehensive. The number and type of professionals involved with a child will depend on their needs at any particular time. Where there is effective interagency collaboration, the needs of the child will be assessed and catered for holistically, allowing the child to progress in

Figure 7.6
Working together for
the child's benefit

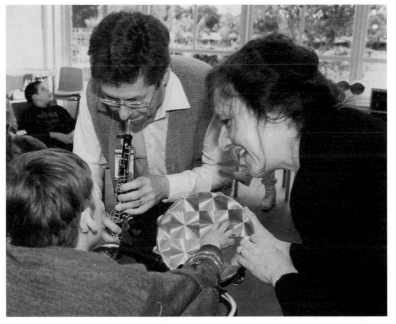

Table 7.1 A chart showing the levels of interagency collaboration compiled using the information provided by the professionals themselves

	Speech Therapist	Educational Pyschologist	Child Care Staff	Physiotherapist	Educational Audiologist	Paediatric Occupational Therapist	Portage Visitor	Senior Medical Technical Officer	School Staff	Parents and Carers
Speech Therapist				×		×	×		×	×
Educational Pyschologist			×	×	×	×			×	×
Child Care Staff		×		×		×			×	×
Physiotherapist	×	×	×			×			×	×
Educational Audiologist		×				×		×	×	×
Paediatric Occupational Therapist	×	×	×	×	×				×	×
Portage Visitor	×									×
Senior Medical Technical Officer					×				×	×
School Staff	×	×	×	×	×	×		×		×
Parents and Carers	×	×	×	×	×	×	×	×	×	

all areas to the best of his or her ability. The discipline of professionals working together is the cornerstone of successful integration of special children into mainstream educational provision. If there is to be a commitment to making integration work, it must start with professionals working together in the best interests of children.

8: AN INCLUSIVE CURRICULUM

Throughout this book we have given significant emphasis to including children with special educational needs in all of the activities on offer within an early years setting. These activities make up part of the whole curriculum. That is everything which goes on within the setting. The whole curriculum also includes the attitude of staff to children and parents, the way that behaviour is managed, the way that individuals are welcomed, the way that people with special needs are portrayed, what is taught and the way things are taught, the way language is used within the taught curriculum and the resources on offer.

The taught curriculum

This might be described as the educational activities and routines used to develop learning. It could be seen as the framework for learning set out by the Qualifications and Curriculum Authority in the Desirable Learning Outcomes. It is also the National Curriculum for Key Stage 1, taught as children enter school.

Access to the curriculum

The aim of including all children within the taught curriculum is a challenging task. It will mean adapting and modifying access to social activities, formal learning situations, and informal day-to-day routines. Should the curriculum be organised in such a way as to take account of a child's special needs, or should the child be given specific support to gain access to the curriculum? The answer is that both should happen. The key question is how.

Unfortunately there is no simple answer to this question. We have to look at examples of good practice, how settings have adapted and changed the curriculum and how staff have developed expertise in supporting children with special educational needs. Such practice seems to have as its core:

- *Collective curriculum planning that, at the outset, considers how all children will be included in activities*
- *A collective view that promotes inclusive education for all children*
- *Staff that have engaged in training to refine and develop their practice in order to identify, observe and support children with special needs*
- *Good communication and trust between staff and parents*
- *Information on policy and procedures regarding special educational needs that is readily available for parents*
- *Assessment, observation and recording procedures that are an integral part of the whole curriculum.*

What is interesting, is that these core features are good practice for *all* settings and for *all* children. They do not specify how to treat an individual child, nor do they identify what to do about a specific condition or disability. That level of refinement will only come when a clear image of the child's strengths and weaknesses has been established and when identification, assessment and planning for individual needs has occurred. All young children should have their early years development monitored in line with the recommendations of the government's Green Paper.

At the moment such monitoring includes:

- *Developmental assessment and screening at clinics and Health Centres*
- *Concern from medical practitioners such as doctors and health visitors*
- *Concern noted by early years staff as part of ongoing assessment*
- *Parental concerns*
- *Baseline Assessment on entry to formal schooling.*

What makes an inclusive curriculum?

The debate as to what makes a good early years curriculum has increased following the introduction of Ofsted inspections for early years settings. The idea of planning in great detail, as required by Ofsted, was new to some providers, although good practice had always included providing a great variety of experiences to stimulate children's learning and development. Ofsted requires providers to work towards achieving the Desirable Learning Outcomes, originally devised by SCAA (now QCA – Qualifications and Curriculum Authority) and the DfEE. An inclusive curriculum will provide a stimulating, but caring and supportive, environment that meets the needs of all children.

Further targets for older children are Baseline Assessment and the Key Stages forming the National Curriculum.

Planning a curriculum

The first stage
Before the formal planning starts, information to answer the following questions is needed:

1. *What do we know about the children's levels of skills, experiences, likes, dislikes?* As a staff team we need to share this information to provide a basis for our planning.
2. *What do we need to know about the children?* To create a curriculum that provides stimulating activities and promotes learning, we need to decide how we will approach record keeping.
   - *What will we keep records about?*
   - *Why are we keeping records?*
   - *How will we use the information?*
   - *How will we gain the information?*
   - *How can we use the information to plan?*

3. *What are our resources?*
   - *equipment*
   - *staff*
   - *parental input*
   - *visitors*

4. *What are our aims?*

What do we want to achieve this year, term, half-term, week? Since we are required to plan for all areas of development, we could use the headings identified in the Desirable Learning Outcomes as a framework for planning. The next step is to identify how planning should happen. Staff team meetings are the ideal setting for this process to take place. The structure, format, order and detail of your plans will be different depending on the needs of children but the fundamental considerations are:

1. *Long term plans*
2. *Short term plans*
3. *Plan evaluation.*

Long term plans

You may decide that topic work should be the basis of your plans. The content of the topics would be linked to all six of the Desirable Learning Outcomes. Tables 8.1 and 8.2 show a topic plan and a format for a daily plan. Table 8.3 shows a more formal approach to planning, this example concentrating particularly on mathematics. Figure 8.1 shows a brainstorm diagram produced during a staff team meeting that took place during the early stages of planning. Care should be taken to ensure that your plans cover the six areas of learning and provide a balanced curriculum overall. How children's progress is to be recorded must also form part of the plans.

Short term plans

The long term plans would then be broken down to provide detailed short term and daily plans. The following considerations need to be highlighted:

- *The needs of the children*
- *How and what the children are going to learn*
- *Staff expertise*
- *Research needed*
- *Budget implications and extra resources*
- *Breakdown of timings*
- *Keyworker system*
- *Staff deployment.*

Plan evaluation

The planning process needs to be continuously evaluated and reviewed. The way this will be done has to be agreed as part of the initial long term plans. Evaluation will provide answers to some of these questions:

- *Are the activities pitched at the right level to interest the children?*
- *Are the children making progress?*
- *Have the children still got time to do what they want to do?*
- *Are we doing too much? too little?*
- *Are we going too fast or slow?*

Remember that there is no point in evaluating your plan if you do not take measures to improve your work when you are not achieving your aims.

Table 8.1 Topic plan

Knowledge and understanding of the world		Creative development	
Nature table with house plants [be aware of safety] Map to be made with children identifying what they saw on outings to form display backdrop.		Collages of natural materials, where possible provided by the children, (seeds, shells, leaves picked up on outings to the seaside and a nature walk) Rest of materials to be used for making a map Children to decorate various containers in which they will plant bulbs.	

Language and Literacy	Theme: Growing Timing: first week		Mathematics
Stories about natural things and growth (*The Little Red Hen*) Rhymes with relevant theme Identify new vocabulary, names of plants and flowers, mathematical measurements Reference books to show stages of plant growth.	Special resources: Bulbs (crocus, miniature daffodils), bulb fibre, beansprouts, carrot tops, containers, mustard and cress seeds, glass container and hyacinth bulb.		Counting opportunities when planting bulbs Chart to measure how long beansprouts, cress take to grow Measuring when filling containers and measuring growth of carrot tops, visual chart to be produced with the children.

Personal and Social development		Physical development	
Talking about growing things Young things need nurturing Children to work in mixed age groups to plant, older ones to be encouraged to help the younger ones.		Music and movement sessions involving starting small and growing Introduce moving against the elements, walking against the wind, sheltering from the rain.	

Table 8.2 Daily plan

Creative		Physical	
Resources:		Resources:	
Staff responsibilities:		Staff responsibilities:	

Language/Literacy	Overall theme:	Knowledge of the World
Resources:	Today's	Resources:
Staff responsibilities:	activities:	Staff responsibilities:

Social/Emotional		Mathematics	
Resources:		Resources:	
Staff responsibilities:		Staff responsibilities:	

Figure 8.1
Brainstorming is a
useful planning tool

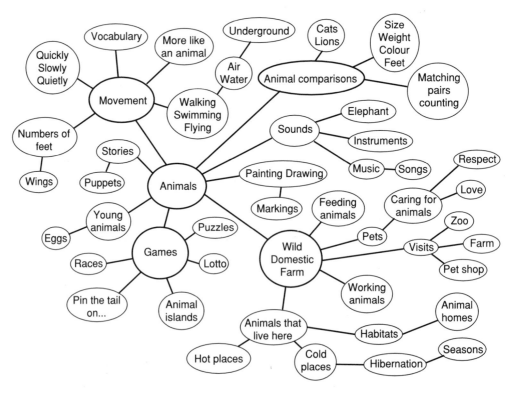

Table 8.3 Curriculum plan

Key Stage 1 reference	Activities	Equipment/resources	Assessment
Select and use appropriate mathematics	Junk modelling [recycling technology], cooking, games, comparisons, matching, sorting	Modelling materials (man made and natural), ingredients, puzzles, games	Observation, questioning, recording
Select and use mathematical equipment and material	Shopping, using money, pattern making, counting, sorting, stories and rhymes	Imaginative play area, till, money, peg boards, tanagrams, specialist manufactured and everyday objects, suitable examples incorporating number	Observation, questioning, recording
Develop different mathematical approach and investigate ways of overcoming difficulties	Measuring and weighing, investigating sand and water, dance	Scales and simple balances, charts and measures appropriate equipment, counting steps	Observation of response
Organise and check their own work	Confirming results, using questions, completing recording documents	Adult confirmation, worksheets	Records products
Understanding of mathematical language	All activities	All resources	Check understanding
Relate numerals and mathematical symbols to a range of situations	Additions and subtraction, sizing, comparisons	Computer, clocks, road signs, worksheets	Product, use language records
Discuss work, respond to and ask mathematical questions	Concepts – full/empty, bigger/smaller	Sand and water equipment, small world play materials, awareness of body parts	Observation, recording, questioning
Use a variety of forms of mathematical presentation	Preparing and using charts, graphs, recording mechanisms, timing	Displays, computers, clocks, timers, sand timer, musical toys	Product recording responses
Recognise simple patterns and relationships, make predictions about them	Drawing, writing, verbal predictions (what will happen), activities to highlight understanding of days of week, weeks in year, seasons	Weather records, diaries, charts, sand and water activities	Product questioning recording

Conclusion

In this chapter we have seen how to plan an inclusive curriculum. The curriculum should be designed so that it will not need to be amended to cater for children with special educational needs. It should be flexible enough to enable *all* children to achieve according to their own individual ability, pace and stage of development. To ensure that providers meet the needs of children with special needs the Code of Practice requires Special Education Plans to be drawn up (see Chapter 3). Such plans identify specific targets and review mechanisms which should enable children to access the inclusive curriculum. These plans are not designed to replace the curriculum.

9: Case Studies

This Chapter is intended to focus in more detail on key issues already discussed in this book. It is presented as a series of case studies which consider:

- The impact of the Code of Practice
- The impact of physical, intellectual and sensory disabilities and learning difficulties on the development of children
- The potential effects of achievement and failure on self-confidence and

self-esteem and methods of encouragement and support
- The central role played by parents in the development of their children
- The need for parents to have all relevant information relating to their children
- Variations in levels of parental involvement and the diversity of family backgrounds
- How to maintain privacy and dignity for the child.

This chapter provides examples of tasks for those undertaking a variety of child care awards which will provide relevant evidence of knowledge and understanding of the issues and practice relating to special education needs. The tasks also provide a useful tool for tutors and others to identify starting points for discussion.

These case studies do not include children who have suffered any kind of abuse. The reason for this is that, although the experience of being abused can have far reaching effects on the child's developmental level and ability to achieve, child abuse in itself is not recognised as a cause of special educational need.

Good practice

To provide for the needs of all children in all early years settings, the framework below can be implemented.

Framework for good practice

1. Management and policies that ensure:
- *All legal requirements of the group are understood and complied with at all times*

- *Employment and management of staff includes*
  - *clear job descriptions*
  - *contracts of employment that set out the rights of both employee and employer*
  - *a staff appraisal system that enables both employees and employers to review all practice*
  - *regular staff planning meetings*
  - *effective deployment of staff*
- *Implementation and review of all policies in operation*
- *Review and update of all prospectuses and other publicity material*
- *Utilisation of all funding methods.*

2. Staff who have the skills to:
- *Promote independence of children*
- *Work with other professionals*
- *Sensitively recognise and respond to the individual needs of children and parents*
- *Support parents and encourage their role as the main educators of their children*
- *Actively support and develop the principles of inclusive education*
- *Work as a SENCO*
- *Plan, design, implement and evaluate an inclusive curriculum*
- *Promote the policies in operation by the setting*
- *Record and use information gathered from observations*
- *Maintain records as agreed with parents.*

3. Curriculum and records that:
- *Ensure each child can develop to their individual potential*
- *Offer a wide range of enjoyable, stimulating activities*
- *Ensure the Desirable Learning Outcomes are being worked towards*
- *Have built in evaluative techniques*
- *Will be shared with and available to parents at all times*
- *Meet the requirements of the Code of Practice.*

4. Resources that:
- *Promote physical access for all children*
- *Include specialist equipment as appropriate to individual needs*
- *Include the use of toy libraries*
- *Promote positive images of all sections of society*
- *Are evaluated and updated wherever possible*
- *Are the best value to be found and make the best use of funds available.*

Case Study

Jamie

Jamie is 1 year old and his mother is considering attending the local Opportunity Playgroup. Jamie was born with a severely inturned left foot and has had two operations to help correct it. He now wears a foot brace to support his foot. This is a very heavy and cumbersome piece of equipment which Jamie hates – he screams every time he sees it.

Jamie is an only child and asks to be carried everywhere although he has been encouraged to try walking. The hospital is very keen for him to walk. He prefers to remain static but will occasionally bottom shuffle towards an object he really wants. He is also unwilling to feed himself. Jamie is reluctant to let his mum out of his sight and makes very loud demanding noises which she correctly interprets. She provides for his needs as quickly as possible and consequently is now showing signs of fatigue and stress. The Opportunity Playgroup supervisor, having talked to his mother during a home visit, has identified the priorities as being:

- *To encourage Jamie and mum to spend some time apart, not only to give his mother a chance to rest but also to encourage Jamie's independence*
- *To encourage Jamie's development of all physical skills*
- *To encourage Jamie to start to use clear words and gesture rather than sounds when he wants something.*

Activity

Suggest three strategies to encourage this child's development. You may like to think about using the Portage method of breaking down tasks into small steps. Your ideas will provide useful evidence for NVQ Unit C17.

Case Study

Ragit

Ragit is 3 years old and has been diagnosed with a congenital heart defect. He will be able to have a corrective operation when he is about 5, but in the meantime his parents have been advised that he can take part in most activities except prolonged physical exertion, so that he does not get out of breath. Ragit is an extremely active little boy who adores all sorts of sports and wants to be running around all the time. He is about to come to your playgroup for three mornings a week.

Activity

What information would you need from Ragit's parents? Think about and describe how you could provide opportunities for Ragit so that he feels integrated in the group.

Case Study

Jemima

Jemima is 1 year old and about to attend a day nursery from 8.00 am to 5.30 pm as her mother wishes to return to full-time work. As far as can be identified at present, Jemima can see large objects and bright colours but cannot follow a finger further than 20 cm from her face.

The nursery has two other babies, aged 3 months and 10 months, being part of a larger unit which cares for 40 children each day. There are also three other children aged between 1 and 2 years. It is planned that Jemima will spend more and more time with them. There is a separate baby room and eating area for the under twos, and a large play room which is well equipped for this age range.

Activity

Your task is to:

- Identify any specialist equipment that would be useful when working with this child
- Identify a list of equipment that you would expect the nursery to have already and highlight any items you feel would not be appropriate for Jemima – give reasons why

> • You are planning to encourage Jemima to become independent and to move around safely. At present she can stand unaided and roll along the floor but has not yet crawled or walked. What agencies would you approach for help?

Case Study

Stacy

Stacy has suffered from asthma and eczema since birth. During the first 3 years of her life, she has suffered several severe asthma attacks (although these are becoming less frequent) and persistent eczema. She has proven allergies to fur, feathers, chocolate and eggs. She is encouraged to take exercise but knows she must stop if she feels breathless. Stacy is a very lively and active little girl. She can, if talked through the process, use her own inhaler. Whilst the asthma seems to be more controlled, the eczema is becoming more of a problem. Her body is often raw in places where skin meets skin, between her fingers and under her arms, for example. The doctor has advised that Stacy should wear cotton gloves whenever possible to provide a barrier, but she does not like them.

Activity

Imagine you are Stacy's main carer and describe her needs to the local Under Fives Group she will be attending next term.

Case Study

Ian

Ian is now $5\frac{1}{2}$ years old. He has attended a village playgroup, spent a term at an Assessment Centre and is now ready to start his first term in mainstream school.

The local health visitor organised Ian's attendance at playgroup as she had concerns about the level of parenting he was receiving at home. He is an only child. His mother was 15 when he was born and his father 19. They have been living in a small council house for the last year. Before this his father was working in a circus and Ian and his mother lived with an elderly aunt. Both parents are illiterate. The health visitor reports that the mother provides meals, but does housework and washing very erratically.

When Ian started the playgroup, his mother bought him for the first session. She said she was not filling in any forms and that the health visitor would deal with all that. The health visitor had arranged to collect Ian and take him home as she was concerned that his mother might forget.

Ian rushed around the group pushing anything and anybody out of his way. He had a permanent smile on his face. He made no sounds at all although he would turn in response to his name. When it was explained to him that certain behaviour was not acceptable, he continued to smile but tried to run off. No activities seemed to engage his attention. Once he had had a quick look at the activities, he started to go through the cupboards until a member of staff physically stopped him.

The staff decided that Ian should be provided with one-to-one attention until he had settled in and understood the rules of the setting. The morning continued in a similar manner with Ian being removed from each activity as he demolished it. When the health visitor arrived the supervisor stated that the group needed help with Ian. This group is held in an old school building and there is a very large area available to the children. The health visitor agreed to support the case for an additional member of staff to support Ian in the group and the group agreed to find an extra volunteer for the sessions in between times. As it happened, Ian did not turn up for the next four sessions. This was reported to the health visitor and Social Services. It was agreed that extra funding for an additional worker would be made available (this level of support is not available in all areas of the county).

After further consultation with the health visitor, it was agreed that Ian's support worker would both collect and take him home as she lived near enough to make this practicable. With this arrangement Ian started to attend more regularly, although he still missed about one in five sessions. When the support worker arrived she would be told he was ill. On two occasions Ian had waved to the support worker from his bedroom and did not appear to have anything wrong with him.

Ian's behaviour during the rest of the term would have remained the same if it had not been for his support worker. She was aware of his problems and able to move quickly to prevent the throwing, pushing, spitting and biting that often occurred. Ian seemed to be most occupied when riding a bike. He did not have this skill when he first came to nursery and shook his head when asked if he had a bike at home. However, once shown what to do he quickly picked up the skill and achieved a great speed on the particular red trike he selected. If he went out to play and this trike was not available, he would scream and try to attack the child who had it. Any adult who intervened was likely to be bitten.

Ian's behaviour continued to cause concern and strategies were introduced to try to minimise the effect! Milk time in the group was communal with everyone sitting down to share a drink and snack. At first Ian would grab as much as he could and run into a corner to eat it. The support worker would keep a very tight hold of Ian when it was announced that the children should have their snacks and drinks. The correct behaviour was shown to Ian at every opportunity and the other children were praised and given extra snacks when they got it right. Ian was told that he could have extras too if he behaved as was expected and after three or four sessions his behaviour improved as long as the support worker was with him. During the rest of the session Ian was still very destructive. He seemed to understand some instructions and definitely understood 'No'.

It was some 2 months before he was heard to say anything. His speech progressed slowly and his level of sentence building was very basic, 'Me want' for example.

The playgroup felt that they needed help and ideas for further strategies to manage Ian's behaviour. By this time some parents had swapped their children from the session Ian attended and others had complained when he had pinched or bitten their children. Although Ian was watched very carefully by his support worker it was difficult to identify when he would be violent as his facial expression remained static and he was also extremely quick.

The county Advisory Teacher attended at the group and observed Ian on three occasions. The outcome of these visits was that Ian was unable to maintain a suitable level of social contact and demonstrated violent behaviour sometimes without provocation. It was agreed that he would benefit from spending some time in an Assessment Centre.

Ian attended the local Assessment Centre in a group of 15 children aged 4 to 11 years. He was put on an individual behavioural management plan that involved a one-to-one worker and rewards for good behaviour. Ian's behaviour gradually improved and his speech was assessed as being only six months behind the expected developmental norm for his age. It was agreed that he could join a speech therapy session already in place at the mainstream primary school he was about to enter.

Activity

Identify how you think this child could best be supported in a reception class with 17 other children.

Case Study

Johab

Johab is 5 years old and has recently moved to Britain from Brunei with his parents, Lily and Keklo. Johab has attended a nursery school whilst in Brunei — see report below. He has now entered Primary School.

Brunei Nursery School, September 1999

This Report was compiled in conjunction with Johab's parents and is confirmed by them as being a joint representation of Johab at this time.

1. Johab experienced difficulties at birth. The umbilical cord caused a part constriction of the airway and resultant minor damage was caused to the brain. Functions of reasoning have, therefore, been delayed and there is also a slight impairment of use of the right side limbs and digits.

2. Johab has attended our school since the age of 2 years, and has built up his time at the school from two morning sessions to full-time provision at $3\frac{1}{2}$ years, at which time his mother returned to part-time day work as a general nurse in the local hospital. His father is an orthopaedic surgeon and also works at the hospital.

3. At 3 years old Johab was assessed by a multidisciplinary team of specialists including pediatrician, teacher, educational psychologist and nursery assistant. This indicated that he had developmental delay and overall was operating at the level of a two-year-old. He was also assessed as having minor difficulty using the right hand side of his body. This results in an uneven gait, and lack of controlled pincer movements with his right hand. It was agreed at this time that Johab would benefit from occupational therapy to encourage the use of his right leg and arm. This has involved various exercises and an emphasis on using both sides of the body together where possible. For example, a great stress has been put on developing

crawling which uses both sides of the body in unison and develops the pathways between the two spheres of the brain. Johab has made limited progress with these exercises and unfortunately does not enjoy them.

4. Johab is smaller than his peers. He is a likeable, attractive child who uses his natural charm to encourage people to do things for him, rather than use his own skills and strength. He had a local nanny at home.

5. A summary of his stage of development on leaving our school:

- Johab enjoys picture books, particularly those with cars or transport in them.

- He uses his left hand to push cars and makes appropriate vroom sounds.

- His speech overall varies in clarity, 'mummy' 'daddy' 'Neja' (his nanny) 'tractor' are very clear and he will attempt most other words when encouraged. He can make his needs known by pointing and if necessary the pointing is accompanied by the word or a sound if he does not know the word. However, we have now found a formula that seems to work – Johab has the reward of a new car when he has learnt another 10 words. His keyworker has been very involved in this initiative and he has dramatically increased his vocabulary over the last 3 months. Sentence formation is still very basic: 'Me want …'.

- He has recently mastered a sit on tractor and although he sometimes tends to make more circular movements to the left, he is using his right leg to move along. These movements are still quite laboured and slower than his peers.

- He responds well to smiles and, although not outgoing, will smile at a child or adult he is not sure of. However, if he does not receive a positive response he will either ignore the other person or move away.

- He makes attempts at recognition of shapes – circle and square are now established, but others are sometimes muddled. He likes red and will recognise and name it, but other colours usually result in the response 'no red'.

- Johab makes an attempt to join in rhymes and particularly likes two rhymes incorporating numbers: 'Baa baa black sheep' and '1,2,3,4,5 Once I caught a fish alive'. He has conceptualised the value of one, two and possibly three.

- Johab doesn't like animals or insects and screams upon sight. He seems to have a real terror of anything, particularly if it moves quickly.

A.J. Knolley, Headmistress

Activity

Given the above information, complete the Entry Profile Sheet for Johab. This information would usually contribute to Baseline Assessment, undertaken at the end of the term after the child's fifth birthday.

Entry Profile Sheet

Child's Name:

Record '1' for each item the child can achieve and '0' for items the child cannot yet achieve.

Reading A: Reading for meaning and enjoyment

1. Holds books appropriately whilst turning the pages and retelling the story from memory ☐
2. Able to predict words and phrases ☐
3. Uses memory of familiar text to match some spoken and written words ☐
4. Reads simple texts ☐

Total ☐

Reading B: Recognition

1. Recognises his or her own name ☐
2. Recognises five letters by shape and sound ☐
3. Recognises 15 letters by shape and sound ☐
4. Recognises all letter shapes by names and sound ☐

Total ☐

Reading C: Phonological awareness

1. Recites familiar rhymes ☐
2. Recognises initial sounds ☐
3. Associates sounds with patterns in rhyme ☐
4. Demonstrates knowledge of sound sequences in words ☐

Total ☐

Writing

1. Distinguishes between print and pictures in his or her own work ☐
2. Writes letter shapes ☐
3. Independently writes own name spelt correctly ☐
4. Writes words ☐

Total ☐

Speaking and listening
1. Recounts events or experiences ☐
2. Asks questions to find out information and listens to the answers ☐
3. Makes up own story and tells it ☐
4. Makes up a story with detail and tells it to a small group and listens to stories ☐
Total ☐

Mathematics A: Number
1. Sorts sets of object by given criterion and explains sorting ☐
2. Counts objects accurately ☐
3. Shows awareness of using addition ☐
4. Solves numerical problems using addition and subtraction ☐
Total ☐

Mathematics B: Using mathematical language
1. Can describe size ☐
2. Can describe position ☐
3. Recognises numbers to 10 and writes 1–10 ☐
4. Can explain an addition sum ☐
Total ☐

Personal and social development
1. Plays collaboratively ☐
2. Is independent and keen to contribute ☐
3. Concentrates without supervision for 10 minutes ☐
4. Expresses own opinions with a range of adults ☐
Total ☐
Grand Total ☐

Case Study

Joane

Joane was born with cerebral palsy. She is now 9 months old and has been receiving support from the Portage Service to encourage her to reach her full potential. She has just learnt to sit up and is now being encouraged to reach for objects. Her plan for the week has been set with the following goals:

Exercises to be repeated five times each for the first 4 days and, if successful, then 10 times each for the last 3 days.

1. Joane to be given an object of interest, either a toy or domestic object, and to be encouraged to explore this object for a short time, whilst an adult talks about it.
2. The object will then be placed just within her grasp and she will be encouraged to retrieve it.
3. The object should be placed slightly further away and Joane encouraged to reach for it.

Praise to be given for all attempts. Objects and toys to be varied to encourage Joane to maintain interest in the activity.

Activity

Make suggestions for next three stages or targets. What do you think would be a realistic timescale for achievement?

Case Study

Pisca

Pisca is now 6 years old and has recently been adopted, having spent his early years in a Romanian orphanage. Nevile and Margaret, his adoptive parents, are investigating local schools and also considering a special school. Pisca's assessments have produced varied results, some saying that integration – possibly with some support – would be the best option, and others saying that with the child's background and learning delay a specialist school is the only option. Whilst his new parents are very anxious for him to achieve his full potential they are reluctant to put him in the position where he might be teased for being different. Physically he is a large child for his age and not very coordinated. Generally he is very amiable unless denied something he really wants. His language was more or less non-existent until about a year ago when Margaret first went to work in the orphanage. He now seems to understand to the level of a 3-year-old, although his speech is stilted and difficult to understand.

Using the Resource Chapter of this Book suggest which organisations could provide further information to enable Pisca's parents to make an informed decision about his education.

Case Study

Katya

Katya is just approaching her fourth birthday and is attending a day care workplace nursery. She has only recently started at the nursery and her keyworker has made the following notes during general observations.

Observation dated 3.3.00

Since starting at the nursery Katya has expressed a liking for the book *Me too* as she has an older sister and the book deals with a younger brother copying his older sibling. This morning Katya selected the book and looked round for an adult to read it to her – there had been a minor injury to another child and all the staff were occupied. I was comforting a new child who wanted a cuddle and reassurance and said I would come over to the book corner as soon as possible. Katya smiled at me and proceeded to look at the book for herself. I observed that she was following the words with her finger and talking quietly. When I was able to get nearer I discovered she was actually reading the story to herself. Once she realised she was being observed she hid the book behind her but continued to smile at me. I sat down with her and asked her where the book had gone and was she enjoying it?

She produced the book and asked me to read it. I said I thought she was reading it. She said, 'No, I want you to read it – if I can't read you will read stories for me. Jemma can read so she doesn't get stories now.' Jemma is Katya's six-year-old sister. I said of course I would read the book but I was interested to know if she could read it. She just shook her head. I read the story to her and then she went off to play with Jo and the cars.

I continued to observe Katya when she was in the book corner. She always checked to see if anyone was watching her and if she saw me she would smile and pat the seat beside her and ask for a story.

Observation 17.3.00

Jo and Katya were playing postmen. Our most recent theme had involved 'people who we see every day' and had included a visit to the local post office where the children had each chosen a picture postcard and written their names and either their own addresses or that of the nursery before posting them at a letterbox. We made a local map showing a photograph of the post office and sorting office, the letterbox, the nursery and some of the children's homes. We played games involving sorting letters — our letters had small photos of the children on them and they chose where to stand in the nursery whilst the 'postman' went round delivering. Since the activity, we have set up a post office counter and designed our own stamps on sticky paper so the children can extend the activity with their own games.

Prior to the observation, Jo and Katya had been busy writing letters and making up envelopes. Katya delivered her letter to Jo and Jo opened it. 'Oh thank you', she said, 'I would love to come to tea on Thursday.' 'No', said Katya, 'it says Friday — tea on Friday at 5.' 'No, Thursday,' said Jo and gave me the letter. 'It's Thursday isn't it?' she asked. I looked at the letter and saw that Katya had written 'Please come to tea on Friday at 5.' The handwriting was very well formed and clearly readable. Katya grabbed the paper back and said, 'We're only playing. You can come on Thursday, Jo.' Katya took Jo's hand and said, 'Let's go and make some cakes.' They both moved off to the playdough table and began to roll out cake shapes.

I had a word with Katya's grandmother who picks her up most days and asked her if Katya could read and write. Grandma stated that she thought Katya was very bright. When reading stories to Katya she had been corrected by her if she got the words wrong. When grandma introduced a game to find the letter K, Katya always got it right. Grandma had extended this game with a few simple words and again Katya was always accurate. However, Grandma was not sure if she was just being lucky in her choices, whether Katya had a good memory, or whether her intellect had advanced to the stage where she was able to read for herself.

Observation 24.4.00

A more formal assessment of Katya's level of development was carried out at the end of the Spring Term. The assessment method involves various games and activities as starting points to record what the child can achieve. We have developed a set of cards to record the child's ability at recognising colour, shape, letters and words. This activity can be used at various levels ranging from very simple colour matching, to matching colour names written in the appropriate colour and colour names in black. We use these cards in a great many different ways which require different levels of achievement. This enables the whole group to feel they are using the same materials and our conclusions can be written to identify the level the child is at. For instance, the starting point for a child of Katya's age would be to identify at least 10 colours in Activity A. We would then progress to see if the child could correctly identify any further colours in Activity B.

- *Activity A: 10 coloured cards set out face up, child asked to find a card with a colour, red for example*
- *Activity B: five further colours are added and the child is asked if they can identify the colour of those cards*
- *Activity C: introducing shapes, the child is asked to find, for example the red triangle*
- *Activity D: matching the written coloured word to the appropriate coloured card*
- *Activity E: matching the black words to the relevant colour*

This form of assessment is used across all six learning outcomes in different ways. For example, to determine physical skills we have cards which identify various movements: able to climb up the climbing frame, hop on one leg 3 times, hop on both legs 3 times. As each activity is confirmed during our normal physical obstacles courses, general inside and outside play, and music and movement sessions the relevant statement is ticked off on the child's records.

My assessment of Katya concluded that she completed all activities in all of the outcomes, except hopping on both legs and catching a ball five times in a row and she was unaware of the names of three objects at the highest level. I feel that this child is extremely well developed for her age and also that she had mastered more than the rudiments of reading and writing. She is wary of acknowledging her skills. This seemed to stem from the fact that she loved having stories read to her and that her older sister is now encouraged to read for herself rather than have stories read to her.

I discussed the position with my supervisor and together we approached Katya's Grandma. Grandma was very interested and felt that Katya should be encouraged in every way. However she returned the next day to say that, having spoken to Katya's parents, they were anxious that she should not be labelled as 'special' or pushed to achieve.

Activity

What sort of advice would you give to the parents to encourage the child to view being able to read as a positive achievement?

Case Study

Gina

Nina works as a Classroom Assistant in a Primary School which is about to welcome the second child of a family. The Petersons have three children – Eric aged 7 is already at the school, Gina aged 5 and Kelvin aged 1 year.

The following information has been made known to Nina:

- Gina has mild spastic cerebral palsy affecting the left side of her body.
- She was involved in an accident 4 months ago when she pulled a kettle lead and ended up with splash burns to her face and chest and severe burns to both thighs and parts of her lower legs. She still has pressure bandages on both legs.
- She is a bright and generally happy child although the injury to her legs has caused her considerable pain and she sometimes gets cross when they hurt.
- Gina has missed out on the last term at nursery because of her injuries. Before this she was working at, or only slightly below the level of her peers. Help was available if Gina requested it, but she is a very independent child and always wanted to do things for herself. However, since her accident she has got used to more help and is reluctant to move about as much as she did because of the pain.
- Her right hand is the preferred one and she loves drawing and colouring and can recognise and write her first name and part of her surname.
- She loves animals and cuddly toys and generally relates well to other children and adults. However she has developed a paranoid fear of people wearing masks or anything on their faces – this might be the result of her hospitalisation.
- Gina's brother Eric is very protective of her and has told her that he will look after her in the playground! The school has had some minor instances of bullying.

Activity

Using the case study complete the chart below.

Gina

List physical needs	List social and emotional needs	List communication needs	List intellectual needs

Overall strategies to support development in these areas

Specific targets with time scales

Case Study

Henry

Henry has been diagnosed with mild autistic tendencies. Comments about him, after half a term in a nursery, including those of his parents, are set out below.

Physical

Henry, at 3 years, is the average size and weight of a 5-year-old. He is uncoordinated and his movements can be unpredictable, particularly when he is tired. He has attacked his keyworker on two occasions when removed from a situation where he was pushing other children, once biting his keyworker and the other time kicking her.

Communication

Speech is still very much at the stage of 'Me do', 'Me want'. Sentence formation is therefore poor for his age. He is quite happy not to communicate at times and will sit staring into space for up to 20 minutes at a time. He will look at books but his concentration span is very limited, usually to no more than 1 minute. He seems attracted by bright colours.

Social and emotional development

Henry does not show pleasure in people's company. He does not enjoy physical contact (cuddles) and will push away other children if they get too near to him. He is still at the stage of solitary play.

Intellectual development

Henry enjoys drawing. He can produce a recognisable house, train and car. He will sit and draw for up to 5 minutes at a time, but generally his concentration span is not more than 2 minutes. He will pick up books but does not start at the beginning and generally flicks through the pages showing no awareness of the order of a book. He does not show interest in construction toys, apart from knocking down structures. He will not attempt to do puzzles of any kind, including simple shape sorters. He does like to play in the water and sand trays but is inclined to become over-excited by the activity. The nursery has decided that they need to assign a specific worker to Henry and to produce an IEP Plan.

Activity

Design an IEP plan for Henry for the coming term.

Case Study

Raising awareness

Paul is an assistant nursery manager in a large workplace nursery. It is his responsibility to organise policy reviews. At present, the nursery has no children with identified special educational needs. He feels that it would be worthwhile to initiate some activities to raise awareness of the issues surrounding special educational needs. His ideas are as follows:

- To include topic work in the nursery that encourages staff and children to look at their own uniqueness.
- Using measurements and charts to show how the group represents a variety of heights, colour of hair, eyes and hand sizes.
- A collage display of my favourite things to include pictures drawn and cut out by the children.
- Topic work on feelings, including fear, with the aim of recognising that when something is unknown it can be threatening.
- Introducing new pictures and posters showing people all over the world, doing different jobs and having different physical and mental capabilities.
- Discussions with the children, utilising their own experiences at all levels: 'Both my mum and dad wear glasses' or 'My granddad only has one leg'. Comments can be built on to encourage children to identify with particular conditions: 'What do you think it feels like if you can't hear properly?'
- Practical exercises such as covering ears and trying to listen or looking through sellotaped glasses.

- Discussion of independence issues. Katy wanted help on the balancing bars, but Joey did not. How would Joey have felt if he had been made to have help? Relate these experiences to people's choices and rights. Someone in a wheelchair may be very happy for you to open a door for them, or they may wish to do it themselves – it is better to ask the person what they want, rather than make an assumption of need.

Activity

How would you monitor the effectiveness of the above ideas? What other suggestions could you make to increase awareness?

Case Study

Patrick

Mark, in his role as a classroom assistant, has been asked by one of the teachers he works with to take particular responsibility for a new child. Patrick is coming into school part way through the summer term. This child is now five years old and has not had experience of any preschool provision. His father has always worked from home and has been his full-time carer. Patrick is described by his father as 'very outgoing, bright but non-conformist'.

Patrick has visited the school on two occasions. The first time he came to join in a PE activity. Patrick would not change his shoes but ran off and attacked all the equipment with gusto, pushing the other children out of the way as he did so – although such pushes were accompanied by a smile and an 'excuse me'. Patrick did not respond when asked to stop or sit down and eventually the teacher took his hand and insisted that he sat down. Patrick then sat and tried to wriggle away to go back to the equipment. The teacher had a word with his father about the need to talk to Patrick about joining in activities and what was expected of him. Patrick's father was not very receptive.

Patrick also came to visit for the last session of an afternoon at storytime. He came in and started to wander round the classroom looking at everything. The teacher invited him over to listen to a story and sit on the floor with the others. Patrick asked what the story was and on being told said, 'Oh, I know that one' and then gave a very good précis of it. The teacher said it would be very nice if he could sit down and listen with the others. Patrick said 'No thanks' and went away again to investigate the classroom. He had just found the LEGO and was beginning to tip it out when the teacher reached him. She asked again for him to join in. Patrick said, 'No, I don't want to – I'd like to play with the LEGO please.'

Activity

What are the issues Mark has to think about in preparation for working with this child.

Case Study

Leanne

Activity

This is an extended case study consisting of various parts. These follow Leanne through from her attendance at playgroup until her assessment at Key Stage 1. After each part you may like to think about how this child's needs were met. Describe anything else that you think could have been done for her. Analyse your own thoughts and feelings about each situation and identify any training that you would need to help you work well with Leanne. Finally, discuss the advantages and disadvantages for Leanne of going to school at the age of 4 years and 1 month.

Part one

Leanne is 3 years old and is just about to start her second term in a busy suburban playgroup. Her keyworker noticed at the end of last term that she did not always answer when spoken to and seemed to be inattentive during story and singing sessions. This was mentioned to her father. He said she had had an ear infection and may have been finding it a little difficult to hear. The doctor was hopeful that, when the infection settled down, Leanne's hearing would improve.

During the planning session for the new term staff discussed Leanne's hearing and it was agreed that her keyworker would monitor her progress. It was decided that, at this time, a special plan for Leanne was not necessary but that the situation would be reviewed at the next meeting in a fortnight's time. The coming half term's theme was 'Textures'. The plan was drawn up with a bias towards enabling 4-year-olds to achieve the Desirable Learning Outcomes, but also to provide activities for younger children to participate in, according to their own level of development.

During the first week, Leanne was still having problems. She was also a bit tearful when leaving dad, who said he thought she had recovered from the ear infection. Leanne was reluctant to settle down in the group and played mostly on her own. Last term she had been very friendly with two other girls and they all spent a lot of time playing in the home corner with the dolls and prams. Leanne now seemed to prefer playing alone with the playdough. She was also reluctant to talk to the adults in the group. Her key-worker spent a lot of time with her but she was unresponsive. The keyworker also noticed that her articulation was indistinct.

Leanne enjoyed making a badge and chose blue velvet as her favourite texture. She liked stroking the badge and nodded when asked if she liked the feel of it. She could not respond when asked to describe how it felt. Given the options of 'smooth', 'soft' and 'rough', Leanne just continued to stroke the material. At the end of the week the key-worker had another word with her father to say that she was concerned that Leanne was having further difficulties with her hearing. Dad said she was fine at home and that she had just got used to being at home with him during the summer. Now she was jealous because her sister was at home with him on her own. Dad works from home and also has a sister living nearby who helps him out. His wife died after giving birth to Bethan, Leanne's younger sister.

Staff agreed that they would identify a number of key situations in which Leanne could be observed in the natural setting of the playgroup. This would allow the observation, however informal, to be valid and reliable.

Activity

Consider how the observation could be implemented.

Part two

At the end of the second week, there was still concern about Leanne's hearing. She responded more to her keyworker but still seemed unwilling to join in group activities.

She appeared not to be listening during circle activities. She very much enjoyed making a puppet – she made a purple dragon, but did not want to make him 'talk' when asked to. She also did not want to be involved in a puppet show during which each child was invited to talk about and to their puppet. She was not as talkative or as clear in her speech as before.

Part three

Leanne was away from playgroup for two weeks. Her father had been in touch to say that she had had another quite severe ear infection and was waiting to see a specialist. When she returned Leanne seemed very withdrawn and cried for her father when he left. She allowed her keyworker to comfort her but didn't want to join in any activities. The keyworker reported this to her father when he collected her. He said he was thinking about keeping her at home for another week. The Supervisor suggested that Leanne's father also contact his health visitor to provide additional professional advice and support.

Part four

The Supervisor of the group received a telephone call from Leanne's father to say that she had been unwell again and that he was keeping her at home. Leanne did not return to playgroup until after the half term break. Her father asked to talk to the keyworker and explained that Leanne was going to be fitted with a hearing aid in the next week. It had been found that she had a 40% hearing loss in one ear and a 10% loss in the other. Her aunt suggested that she could attend one session a week with Leanne. The group, at this stage, made a note of concern and placed Leanne at Stage 1 of the Code of Practice. He father was fully consulted and agreed that this step should be taken in accordance with the policies of the group.

Part five

Leanne was kept at home during the remainder of the half term. She had had her hearing aid fitted, but regularly turned it off. During this time Leanne had two visits from her keyworker with three of her playgroup friends. Everyone helped to make a large card and they took photographs of the activities that been been going on in the group. The keyworker also gave Leanne's father the names and addresses of the local representatives for the RNID, who provide support and materials for staff and parents.

Evaluate the Individual Educational Plan designed for Leanne. Describe how you would work with her if you were her keyworker, the systems you would introduce to feedback information to her father and how you would propose to work with Leanne's aunt.

Part six

At the next Staff Team Meeting the following decisions and plans were made relating to Leanne:

- Her keyworker would work with Leanne on a one-to-one basis initially for the first week and then as needed.
- Leanne's aunt and the keyworker would meet to discuss how she could help.
- It was agreed that the aunt would stay during the first session to reassure Leanne, but would try to encourage Leanne's independence as much as possible. She would encourage Leanne to go to her keyworker with any problems.
- Encouraging Leanne's independence in all areas was a priority. Leanne had begun to ask for help in toileting and other areas, where as before she had been very able to manage herself.
- Health would be the next topic to be covered as Leanne tended to react badly when confronted by nurses and doctors. The keyworker suggested that a positive approach be used. Leanne would be encouraged to talk about her experiences and would be seen as the expert on hospitals.
- An Individual Educational Plan would be prepared for Leanne and progress would be discussed in a meeting between Dad, aunt, keyworker and supervisor on a fortnightly basis.

The priority issues were:

- *to ensure Leanne settled back into the group as quickly as possible*
- *to re-establish the relationship between Leanne and her keyworker with support from the aunt*
- *to encourage and enable Leanne to re-establish relationships with the other children*
- *to ensure that the other children were aware of Leanne's hearing impairment and how it would affect her communication with them*

- to ensure that Leanne was encouraged to take part in all activities and not to use her hearing difficulties as a barrier.

At the review of the above plan it was agreed by all that Leanne was beginning to settle down again. She had slowly begun to build relationships with her peers and had been observed watching the same three girls on four occasions. The keyworker felt that she had also confirmed her relationship with Leanne. She had also encouraged Leanne to go to the toilet on her own, although the aunt reported that she still asked for assistance at home occasionally. Leanne had joined in the discussions about her visits to hospital but only responded to the closed questions and declined to answer any open questions about her experiences. She had been encouraged to talk at every opportunity but was still only responding with monosyllables, or just shaking her head whenever asked anything requiring a longer response.

Part seven

By the end of April Leanne had been offered a place in the local primary school reception class as part of the general intake in September. Leanne's father spoke to the school staff about her hearing difficulties and was advised that she should be able to cope. There will be 28 children in the class for the coming term with the assistance of a non-teaching assistant for four mornings a week. This will rise to about 37 in the following term, by which time the first intake should have settled. The supervisor of the playgroup was concerned that Leanne would not fit in at school. She was still very unsure of herself and had not made any effort to mix socially with the other children. She was still not using her hearing aid all the time and was physically quite weak. Leanne was away from the group with further ear infections for five out of the eight weeks of her last term.

Part eight

As Leanne had very limited access to the group she was not able to join in all the activities that were designed for the 4-year-olds to help them towards achieving the Learning Outcomes.

The Playgroup's assessment forms were completed by the keyworker using the key set out below, and following discussion with Leanne's father and aunt.

Key

a = insufficient evidence to comment
b = assumed from limited observation
c = confirmed – consistent achievement
d = not yet achieved

Personal and social development

Can leave carer without distress	d
Has established relationship with adult/s	c
Has established relationship with other children	d
Is responsible for own toileting	c
Understands need for hygiene	a
Asks questions to solve problems	a
Understands and can illustrate a variety of feelings	a
Understands right and wrong	c
Takes part in games and takes turns/shares as directed	a
Takes part in games and awaits turn	a
Understands people come in a wide variety of ages, sizes, colours etc.	a
Understands the needs of living things and respects such needs	c

Language and literacy

Understands how books work – that they go from top to bottom, left to right, and that the written word relates to what the story says	b
Enjoys stories – in small and large groups	d
Can relate stories back to an adult	d
Takes part happily in role play/drama	d
Knows a number of nursery rhymes, songs and poems	d
Makes up own story/scrapbooks	d
Recognises own name and can write some or all of it, using upper and lower case letters as appropriate	b
Recognises familiar words	a
Recognises some letters	a
Knows the name and sound of letters	a
Increases vocabulary all the time	d
Can recognise rhymes and rhyming sounds e.g. cat, mat, sat, fat	a

Knowledge and understanding of the world

Can identify and name close family members	b
Understands wider family – grandparents, aunts, uncles etc.	a

Can recall and describe events they have experienced, e.g. holidays, Christmas, birthdays etc. — a

Can recognise and describe features of living things — a

Can identify sequences — a

Can describe and recognise features of the area in which they live — a

Can select relevant materials and take part in activities involving: — b

Cutting, holds scissors correctly, cuts straight single cut, cuts more complicated shapes — b

Joining — b

Folding, can recognise that a paper shape is now smaller and count sections — b

Junk modelling, can select and describe actions, materials and sometimes end product — b

Uses a range of construction toys — a

Recognises technological machines, e.g. computers, telephones etc. — a

Mathematics

Recognises and can name various shapes: circle, rectangle, triangle, square — a

Can sequence/describe in a variety of ways: small/bigger/biggest, tadpole to frog, breakfast, lunch, tea etc. — a

Recognises and can recreate patterns — b

Can make sets of ... — b

Understands and can describe a variety of concepts: behind/in front, up/down, over/under — a

Recognises written numbers 1–10 and can count to at least 10. — a

Understands that adding will increase number and taking away will decrease — a

Can give examples of numbers in everyday use: knows house number, telephone number, etc. — b

Can record numbers — b

Creative development

Describes the shape of objects, e.g. windows, doors, box etc. — a

Participates and describes reactions to a variety of textures — b

Participation in activities using widest possible variety of materials: various thicknesses and types of paint, paper, brushes, felt tips, pens, pencils, pastels, charcoal etc. — c

Participates and describes reactions to a variety of sounds — a

Takes part and can predict results when combining substances, e.g.
mixing colours, melting, mixing cooking ingredients   a

Can make up stories and take part in imaginative play   a

Joins in music/dance/movement sessions and can describe their actions and
demonstrate feeling, e.g. by using gentle movements to soft music, heavy
movements to loud   d

Physical development

Small manipulative control: Using scissors, holds correctly, makes single
straight cut, attempts more complicated shape, always cuts accurately   c

Pencil control: holds pencil correctly in chosen hand with constant preference,
makes meaningful marks, can follow patterns, can produce recognisable face,
figure, house   c

Large gross movements:

Overall coordination   a

Moves in time to music   a

Can catch a large ball sometimes, often   a

Can catch small ball sometimes, often   a

Can catch bean bag sometimes, often   a

Can throw above sometimes, often at target   d

Can kick large ball with one foot or both
feet, i.e. left and right – not together!   d

Can hop as above   d

Can jump with feet together   d

Can jump straddled   d

Can skip   d

Can pedal a trike or bike forwards   d

Can pedal a trike or bike backwards   d

Moves with confidence on large equipment or obstacle course   d

Can describe movements in terms of concept, e.g. down the slide, through the
tunnel   d

Takes part in simple team games and races   d

Shows awareness of space, recognises how much room they need to move in a
specific way   d

Part Nine

Leanne is now a term and a half into her school life. Baseline Assessment was undertaken 6 weeks into her school career – see below:

Baseline Assessment

Individual Record Sheet

Child's Name: Leanne
Record '1' for each item the child can achieve and '0' for items the child cannot yet achieve.

Reading A: Reading for meaning and enjoyment
1. Holds books appropriately whilst turning the pages and retelling the story
   from memory   1
2. Able to predict words and phrases   0
3. Uses memory of familiar text to match some spoken and written words   0
4. Reads simple texts   0
Total   1

Reading B
1. Recognises his or her own name   1
2. Recognises five letters by shape and sound   1
3. Recognises 15 letters by shape and sound   0
4. Recognises all letter shapes by names and sound   0
Total   2

Reading C: Phonological awareness
1. Recites familiar rhymes   1
2. Recognises initial sounds   0
3. Associates sounds with patterns in rhyme   0
4. Demonstrates knowledge of sound sequences in words   0
Total   1

Writing
1. Distinguishes between print and pictures in his or her own work   1
2. Writes letter shapes   1
3. Independently writes own name spelt correctly   1
4. Writes words   0
Total   3

Speaking and listening
1. Recounts events or experiences   1
2. Asks questions to find out information and listens to the answers   0

3. Makes up own story and tells it 0

4. Makes up a story with detail and tells it to a small group and listens to stories 0

Total 1

Mathematics A: Number

1. Sorts sets of object by given criterion and explains sorting 1

2. Counts objects accurately 1

3. Shows awareness of using addition 0

4. Solves numerical problems using addition and subtraction 0

Total 2

Mathematics B: Using mathematical language

1. Can describe size 1

2. Can describe position 0

3. Recognises numbers to 10 and writes 1–10 1

4. Can explain an addition sum 0

Total 2

Personal and social development

1. Plays collaboratively 0

2. Is independent and keen to contribute 0

3. Concentrates without supervision for 10 minutes 0

4. Expresses own opinions with a range of adults 0

Total 0

Leanne had three more ear infections and her hearing has gone down to 30% in one ear and 35% in the other. She has been fitted with hearing aids for both ears. She has been away for a total of seven weeks during her school life.

Her teacher thinks that Leanne could benefit from extra support to bring her up to the standard of the other children and has advised that her father approach the authorities and ask for Leanne to be statemented. Leanne's teacher describes her present developmental stage as being:

Leanne was still at stage 2 of the reading scheme the class was using whilst the rest of the class were mainly achieving stages 4 and 5. The norm would be stage 4 for this age group. Her vocabulary and pronunciation of words was considerably behind that of her peers. She spent time looking at books and when asked would make a good attempt at describing the storyline. This seemed to be based on the pictures rather than on recognising words.

Leanne was reluctant to join in physical activities – her balance was not good due to the problems with her ears and she was very unsure of trying out equipment or moving to music. She was very good at cutting out and drawing and her artistic skills are among the best in the class. She was also good with clay and anything involving small motor movements.

Leanne seemed to enjoy taking part in science experiments but she was not good at expressing her thoughts verbally. She did not offer solutions to problems, although she often nodded to agree with a correct solution.

Overall Leanne was still finding it difficult to mix with the other children – as she had had so much time off, friendships were difficult to form and the other children often became frustrated when trying to communicate with her. They tended not to give Leanne time to assimilate what was going on and to formulate her responses. She became a loner and was teased by some of the children – consequently her self-esteem was low and she was very reluctant to try anything new as she thought she would fail. Her academic potential was difficult to assess as she had problems expressing herself, apart from through art.

On the Section of the Local Authority form asking for parents to contribute their views to the statementing process Leanne's father wrote:

'Leanne has suffered with her hearing from the age of two. At first it was thought that the ear infections she had were only those normal to childhood, but unfortunately they got worse and her hearing suffered as a result of severe infections. Leanne has also gone through the trauma of losing her mother when she was just two years of age. My sister lives near us and has supported me greatly with both children. Leanne has a sister a year younger than her, Bethan. Leanne asks questions about her mother but as she was so young does not seem to miss her as a person. I have worked from home since my wife's death and have always been able to ensure a stable and supportive home life for both girls.

Leanne's hearing problems have slowed down her development in other areas. Before the problems became severe she was developing in line with her peers. Missing playgroup and school time have meant that she is now unsure of making personal relationships which are further impaired by her hearing difficulties. She has a very good and positive relationship with my sister and myself, and is developing a close relationship with her maternal grandmother who has recently returned from living abroad. Leanne also enjoys her sister's company and they play together mostly very amiably.

I feel that Leanne would benefit greatly from extra help with reading and communication, perhaps with speech therapy, which has now been suggested by her specialist. I also feel that she needs reassurance to enable her to develop relationships with other children and adults. She has become reluctant to mix with the other children as she was teased about her hearing aids and called "stupid" and "clumsy" because she could not use the PE balancing equipment. I have spoken to her teacher about this and have been reassured that appropriate action was taken, but I have yet to see evidence that things have improved.'

Following the collection of evidence from the school, Leanne's father, Leanne's GP and specialist, a statement was issued. This said that Leanne should receive three half-hour support periods to support her communication development. In practice this meant that she attended a joint speech therapy session with three other children. This was coordinated by a speech therapist who visited the school approximately twice each half term and agreed a programme for individual children. This was carried out by a non-teaching assistant in a separate area once a week. During the other two sessions, Leanne worked with a class assistant on a one-to-one basis. This involved additional reading support and work with phonics to improve Leanne's communication skills. Her father also obtained some information about lip reading and worked at home to encourage Leanne to develop this skill. Leanne's teacher did some work with the whole class raising awareness of a wide variety of physical impairments with the emphasis on building an inclusive and supportive society. Consequently, the teasing stopped and the teacher encouraged Leanne during PE lessons, without applying pressure, and praising her at all times for her efforts.

Part ten

The first review of the statement concluded that Leanne's level of support should continue without amendment. Leanne continued to make consistent progress.

At this time Leanne's achievements at school in English were equivalent to Level 1 in Key Stage 1 – that is she was able to use everyday words to describe things she was interested in. She was trying hard to listen and understand what was said to her, however teachers and class assistants had to be very aware to check her understanding. Leanne was reluctant to speak in class, but was able to explain her ideas and concepts on a one-to-one basis given sufficient time and encouragement to do so.

Leanne was placed at Level 1 for most of this Attainment Target, which would be normal for her age. Her class statistics are:

> Level 1 = 7 pupils
> Level 2 = 23 pupils
> Level 3 = 5 pupils
> Level 4 = 2 pupils

Activity

Assess the support given to this child and identify any changes you feel would have been beneficial.

Figure 9.1a

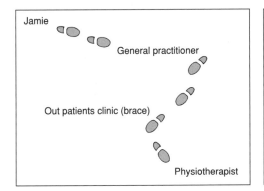

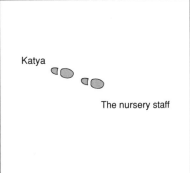

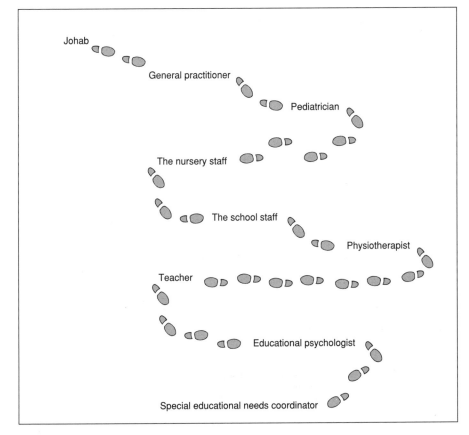

Figure 9.1b

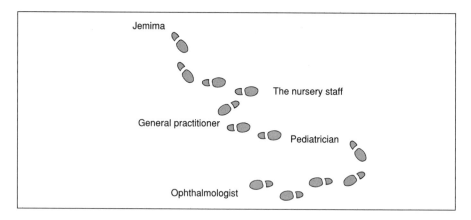

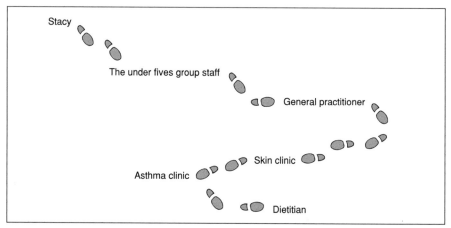

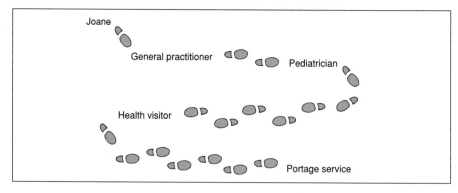

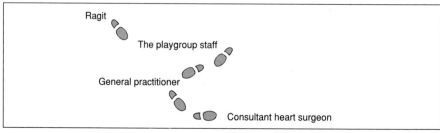

Figure 9.1c

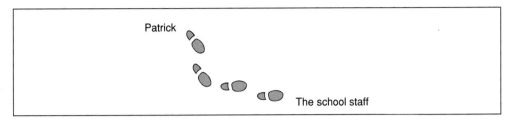

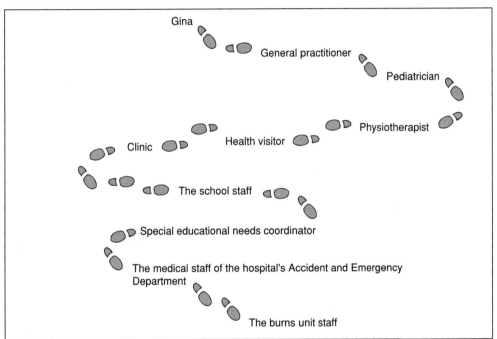

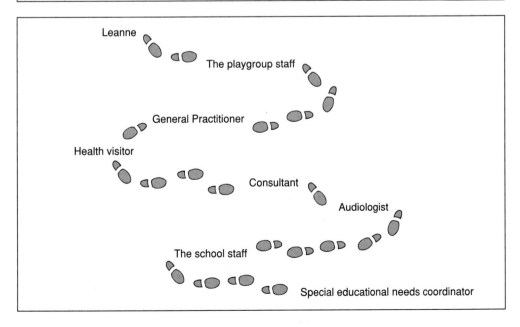

Figure 9.1d

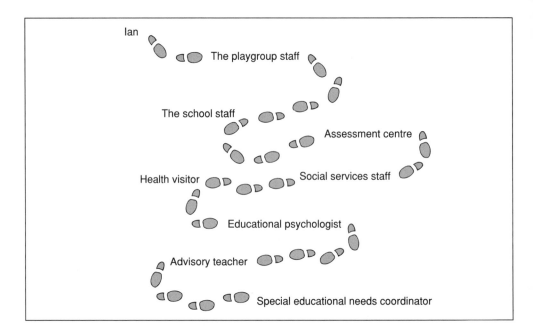

FURTHER READING

Your course tutor may also suggest books for you to read.

BOOKS

Association of Metropolitan Authorities (1994) *Special Needs – Services for Children with Disabilities*.

Dare, A. and O'Donovan, M. (1997) *Caring for Young Children with Special Needs*, Stanley Thornes Publishers Ltd.

Department for Education and Employment (1994) *Code of Practice on the Identification and Assessment of Special Educational Needs*.

HMSO (1991) *The Children Act Guidance and Regulations Volume 6 Children with Disabilities*.

Hobart, C. and Frankel, J. (1994) *A Practical Guide to Child Observation* Stanley Thornes Publishers Ltd.

NSPCC (1994) *Protecting Children: A Guide for Teachers*.

Shar, R. (1995) *The Silent Minority: children with disabilities in Asian families* (Second Edition) National Children's Bureau.

JOURNALS

Special Children
British Journal of Special Education
Child Language Teaching and Therapy

EDUCATIONAL PRESS

Times Educational Supplement

APPENDIX 1

Abbreviations

These are some definitions that you may come across during your studies.

DfEE   Department for Education and Employment
EBD   Emotional and Behavioural Difficulties
EDP   Education Development Plan
EP   Educational Psychologist
EYDP   Early Years Development Plan
FE   Further Education
FEFC   Further Education Funding Council
GCSE   General Certificate of Secondary Education
GNVQ   General National Vocational Qualification
GO   Government Office
HMI   Her Majesty's Inspector
ICT   Information and Communications Technology
IEP   Individual Education Plan
IT   Information Technology
ITT   Initial Teacher Training
LEA   Local Education Authority
LMS   Local Management of Schools
LSA   Learning Support Assistant
NCET   National Council for Educational Technology
NHS   National Health Service
NQT   Newly Qualified Teacher
NRA   National Record of Achievement
NVQ   National Vocational Qualification
OFSTED   Office for Standards in Education
OHMCI   Office of Her Majesty's Chief Inspector
PRU   Pupil Referral Unit
QCA   Qualifications and Curriculum Authority
SEN   Special Educational Needs
SENCO   Special Educational Needs Coordinator
TTA   Teacher Training Agency

APPENDIX 2

Statements

For children with complex needs, statements fulfil three main functions. They are part of the ongoing support available to children and parents and help to define:

1. *What are the child's needs*
2. *The provision to meet those needs*
3. *Who will do what to support the child.*

At any one time almost 233,000 pupils (almost 3% of the school population) have the protection of a statement. When the Code was introduced, it was envisaged that the needs of the majority of children with SEN would be met by its school-based stages.

The number of children with statements has been steadily rising:

1991	*153,228*
1992	*160,759*
1993	*178,029*
1994	*194,541*
1995	*211,307*
1996	*227,324*
1997	*232,995.*

The growth has been most marked in mainstream primary and secondary schools, where numbers of pupils with statements more than doubled from 62,000 in January 1991 to 134,000 in January 1997. The process takes time, is costly and places families under considerable strain.

APPENDIX 3

Support services

This appendix gives sources for information about conditions that may have an educational implication for children and carers.

Special thanks to Avril Cox who assisted in the preparation of this information.

Arthritis
Arthritic Association
First Floor
2 Hyde Gardens
Eastbourne
Sussex
BN21 4PN
Telephone: 01323 416550

Asthma
National Asthma Helpline
Telephone: 0345 010203

Attention deficit hyperactivity disorder
ADD Information Services
PO Box 340
Edgeware
Middlesex
HA8 9HL
Telephone: 020 8905 2013

Family Support Group
1a The High St
Dilton Marsh
Nr Westbury
Wiltshire

BA 13 4DL
Telephone: 01373 826045

Autism and Asperger syndrome
National Autistic Society
393 City Rd
London
EC1 1NE
Telephone: 020 7833 2299

Autism Helpline
Telephone: 020 7903 3555

Blindness
Royal National Institute for the Blind
224 Great Portland Street
London
W1N 6AA
Telephone: 020 7388 1266

National Federation of the Blind UK
Unity House
Smythe Street
Westgate
West Yorkshire
WF1 1ER
Telephone: 01924 291313

Brittle bones disease
Brittle Bone Society
30 Guthrie St
Dundee
Scotland
DD1 5BS
Telephone: 01382 204 446/7

Cerebral palsy
SCOPE
The Anderson Centre
Spitfire Close
Ermine Business Park
Huntington
Cambridgeshire
PE18 6YB

Cerebral Palsy Helpline
Telephone: 0800 626216

Cystic fibrosis
Cystic Fibrosis Trust
Alexandra House
5 Blythe Rd
Bromley
Kent
BR1 3RS
Telephone: 020 8464 7211

Deafness
National Deaf Children's Society
15 Dufferin St
London
EC1Y 8PD
Telephone: 020 7250 0123

Royal National Institute for the Deaf
19–23 Featherstone St
London

EC1Y 8SL
Telephone: 202 7296 8000

Diabetes
British Diabetic Association
10 Queen Street
London W1M OBD
Telephone: 020 7323 1531

Down's syndrome
Down's Syndrome Association
155 Mitcham Rd
London
SW17 9PG
Telephone: 020 8682 4001

Dyslexia
British Dyslexia Association
98 London Rd
Reading
Berks
RG1 5AU

Helpline
Telephone: 01734 66871

Dyspraxia
Dyspraxia Trust
8 West Alley
Hitchen
Herts
SG5 1EG
Telephone: 01462 454986

Epilepsy
British Epilepsy Association
Anstey House

40 Hannover Square
Leeds
LS3 1BE
Helpline
Telephone: 0800 309030

Hemiplegia

Hemi-Help
166 Boundaries Rd
London
SW12

HIV

ADVERT (Aids Education Research Trust)
11–13 Deene Parade
Horsham
West Sussex
RH12 1JD
Telephone: 01403 210202

Huntington's disease

Huntington's Disease Association
108 Battersea High St
London
SW11 3HP
Helpline
Telephone: 01924 280062

Hydrocephalus

Association for Spina Bifida and
Hydrocephalus
ASHBA House
42 Park Rd
Peterborough
PE1 2UQ
Telephone: 01733 555985

Hyperactivity

63 Arundel Rd
Littlehampton
West Sussex
Telephone: 01903 725182

Leukaemia

The Leukemia Care Society
14 Kingfisher Rd
Venny Bridge
Pinhoe
Exeter
Devon
EX4 8JN
Telephone: 01392 464848

Muscular dystrophy

Muscular Dystrophy Group
7–11 Prescott Place
London
SW4 6BS
Telephone: 020 7720 8055

Sickle cell anemia

Sickle Cell Society
54 Station Rd
London
NW10 4UA
Telephone: 020 8961 7795

Speech and language disorders

ICAN Barbican Citygate
1–3 Dufferin St
London
EC1Y 8NA
Telephone: 020 7374 4422

AFASIC
347 Central Markets
Smithfield
London
EC1A 9NH
Telephone: 020 7236 3632

Spina bifida
ASBAH
ASBAH House
41 Park Rd
Peterborough
PE1 2UQ
Telephone: 01733 555988

Spinal injury
Spinal Injury Association
76 St James Lane
London
N10 3DF
Telephone: 020 8444 2121

Support/advice
Network 81
1–7 Woodfield Terrace
Chapel Hill
Stanstead
Essex
CM 24 8AJ
Telephone: 01279 647415

Tourettes syndrome
Tourettes Syndrome Association
169 Wickham Street
Welling
Kent
DA16 3BS

Tuberous sclerosis
Tuberous Sclerosis Association
Little Barnsley Farm
Milton Rd
Cats Hill
Bromesgrove
Worcs
B61 0NQ
Telephone: 01527 871898

MOVE

MOVE stands for Mobility Opportunities Via Education. It is an instructional programme used by teachers, therapists, parents and carers to help learners with severe disablities to sit, stand and walk. These skills lead to a much fuller participation in daily learning and activity. The programme is designed for use with children and young people.

For further information contact:

MOVE International (Europe)
University of Wolverhampton
Gorway Road
Walsall WS1 3BD

MOVE Equipment catalogue
Rifton
Darvell
Robertsbridge
East Sussex
TN32 5DR

PLANET
c/o Harperbury Hospital
Harper Lane
Radlett
Herts
WD7 9HQ

NPFA
25 Ovington Square
London
SW3 1LQ
Telephone: 020 7584 6445
Fax: 020 7581 2402

Child Accident Prevention Trust
4th Floor
Clerks Court
18–20 Farringdon Lane
London
EC1R 3AU
Telephone: 020 7608 2838
Fax: 020 7608 3674

National Play Information Centre (NPIC)
359–361 Euston Road
London
NW1 3A1
Telephone: 020 7383 5455
Fax: 020 7387 3152

Pre-school Learning Alliance
61–63 Kings Cross Road
London
WC1X 9LL
Telephone: 020 7833 0991

National Centre for Play
Moray House College of Education
Holyrood Road
Edinburgh

EH8 8AQ
Telephone: 0131 556 8455

National Association for Children in Hospital
Argyle House
29/37 Euston Road
London
NW1 1LT
Telephone: 020 7629 8361

Play Matters/Active (National Toy Libraries Association)
68 Churchway
London
NW1 1LT
Telephone: 020 7387 9592

Disability Now
12 Park Crescent
London
W1N 4EQ
Telephone: 020 7636 5020

National Library for the Handicapped Child
University of London
20 Bedford Way
London
WC1E 0AL

Contact-A-Family
16 Strutton Ground
London
SW1P

National Deaf Blind and Rubella Association
311 Grays Inn Road
London
WC1

National Society for Mentally
Handicapped Children and Adults
(MENCAP)
123 Golden Lane
London
EC1Y

Kith and Kin
c/o Maurice Collins
6 Grosvenor Road
Muswell Hill
London
N10

There are many more societies at national, regional and local level. Your local library, Council for Voluntary Service/Community Service, Rural Community Council and Citizens' Advice Bureau should be able to put you in touch with local societies and also local branches of national bodies. Social Services will have a list of special playgroups and play projects in your area, and details of all kinds of aids, services, facilities and resources. Some local bodies publish directories of resources and services for people with disabilities. The DfEE Code of Practice: Guide for Parents is also worth consulting. Details of all state benefits can be obtained from the Citizens' Advice Bureau or your local Department of Social Security.

APPENDIX 4

The Internet

The Internet is a great source of information on special educational needs. The volume of information is vast: from small Web Pages created by individuals focussing on specialist areas to large Web Sites, which cover many separate aspects of special education. Many voluntary sector groups and parent support groups are also represented. All can be accessed via a computer which is connected to the Internet. You may have one at home. Alternatively, try your college or local library.

Examples of some of the Web Pages on offer can be seen on the following pages. The selection here represents a tiny proportion of all the Web Sites on offer, but they will give you a flavour of what to expect. There are also interactive Web Sites that allow educationalists and parents to communicate with each other from computers all over the world. You may also care to access the Open Government Web Site, where you will find up to date Government Reports including those related to special education.

SOME USEFUL ADDRESSES ON THE WEB

Try (via search) 'Inclusive Technology' and 'Schoolzone'. Both are excellent web sites for special needs.
Open Government Information (DfEE):
http://www.hmso.gov.uk/acts/acts1996/96056-zd.htm
Government information on special educational needs. The DfEE also have a web page and you can download to disk government reports and consultation papers. A very good way of gaining lots of information.

Special Educational Needs and Information Technology:
http://www.nfer.ac.uk/pubs/special.htm
Based on case studies of ten pupils, this report presents a range of strategies which have been found to be effective by teachers and support staff in the use of information technology with pupils with special educational needs in mainstream schools.

NASEN:
http://www.littleheath.essex.sch.uk/useful.htm
The National Association for Special Educational Needs (NASEN) is a national charity whose aim is to promote the education, training, advancement, development and treatment of all infants, children, young persons and others of whatever age with special educational needs or learning difficulties.

The British Dyslexia Association:
http://www.bda-dyslexia.org.uk/d03parents/p03edact.htm

SENCO Information:
http://www.becta.org.uk/projects/senco/senit/senit.html
The SENCO Information Exchange covers special educational needs issues which are current and which are of interest to all those working in the field. Amongst other items, you will find information about the NCET SENCO project, contents pages of a range of special needs journals and information about recent reports relating to SEN.

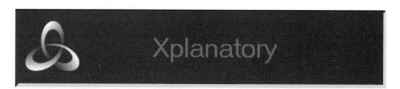

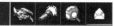

References and resources

 Xplanatory: References and Sources
Here follows a list of recent references and sources on a range of Special Educational Needs

(Key texts, which are usually course readers, have this icon next to them)

- Adults with Special Needs
- ADD/ADHD
- Assessment
- Advocacy
- Autism & Asperger Syndrome
- Biographical Accounts
- Bullying
- Challenging Behaviour
- Circles
- Classroom Assistants
- Code of Practice
- Curriculum Change
- Differentiation
- Dyspraxia
- Emotional Behavioural Difficulty
- Fiction & SEN

- Handwriting
- Hearing Impairment
- Historical and Contemporary Issues
- I.T. & Special Needs
- Individual Education Plan
- Inclusion
- Information Technology
- Language and Communication
- Learning Difficulties
- Management & Special Needs
- Medical Conditions
- Multi-Sensory Impairment
- The Nature and Development of Mind
- OFSTED
- Parent Teacher Partnership

- Personal Construct Psychology
- Physical Disability
- Psychological Perspectives
- Readability
- Research Methods
- S.E.N. in Further Education
- S.E.N. in Higher Education
- S.E.N. in Primary Schools
- S.E.N. in Secondary Schools
- S.E.N. Legislation
- Severe Learning Difficulties
- Self Esteem
- Specific Learning Difficulties
- Spelling
- Thinking Skills
- Visual Impairment and Blindness

This Page was created by the S.N.R.D.C. Please send any comment to: M.Blamires@cant.ac.uk

Somerset Education Services

Support for Parents and Children

Special Educational Needs	Pupil and Student Services
Special Education Service	Pupil and Student Services
BehaviourSupport Services	• Pupil Support Team
Education Psychology Service	• School Transport
Hearing Support Service	• Parent Liaison Service
Learning Support Services	• Student Grants
Physical Disability Support Service	• Early Years
Parents' Forums	Parentline Helpline

Special Educational Needs

- Special Education Service
- BehaviourSupport Services
- Education Psychology Service
- Hearing Support Service
- Learning Support Services
- Physical Disability Support Service
- Parents' Forums

Pupil and Student Services

Pupil and Student Services

- Pupil Support Team
- School Transport
- Parent Liaison Service
- Student Grants
- Early Years

Parentline Helpline

Student Grants

- Support for Students in Higher Education (1998/99 to 1999/2000 and beyond)
- Mandatory Student Support for Higher Education 1998/99
- Mandatory Student Support for Higher Education 1999/2000
- Discretionary Student Grants
- Student Travel 1998/99
- 16+ Travel for Students with Special Needs, Disabilities and Medical Problems

SchoolTransport

- School Transport Code of Good Practice

Starting School

Parentline Helpline
8.30 am-5.00 pm weekdays
0845 6045555

Top of this page

Somerset Education Services
Home Page

Somerset Home Page

This information was last updated: 19 October 1998

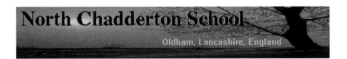

Department of Individual Studies

Head of Department : Mrs.G.Jones

Special Needs Resources

- ADD/ADHD European Home Page
- Special Educational Needs (NGfL site)
- Special Educational Needs Sservice in Swansea (SENS)
- Centre for the study of Autism
- Children and Adults with Attention Deficit Disorder
- Childrens Education
- Center for New Discoveries in Learning
- Communciation Aids for Language and Learning
- Cool Safe Linksfor kids, parents and teachers
- DownsNet Home Page
- Dyslexia : special needs
- Instant Access Treasure Chest
- Marc's Special Education Page
- Special Education Resources on the Internet (SERI)
- Special Needs Bibliography
- The Maddux Special Education Homepage

Asperger's Syndrome/ Disorder

One of our students, Matthew Saberi, gives and introduction to Asperger's Syndrome, and he provides links to sites which give further details and information . Matthew will be reviewing some of the sites he has visited .

Introduction to Asperger's Syndrome

Learning Styles

- Assessing Your Learning Style
- Learning Styles (1)
- Learning Styles (2)

Gifted Child Resources

- Characteristics of the Gifted Child
- The Gifted Child Society
- Helping Your Highly Gifted Child
- The young gifted child at school

Return to Homepage

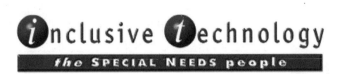 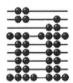

Special Needs Articles
Special Needs Information
Search and Site Index
Catalogue
Contact Inclusive Technology
Making the most of the Inclusive website

Enabling Education Network
ISEC 2000
Octopus Web Site Preview
Site Report from Webtrends

 **April 1999 Updates**

 leave your comments in our guestbook

Inclusive Writer Review - Fiona Sanderson reviews Inclusive Writer - **the** pictorial word processor
ONSEC '99 - SEN Conference - a national conference examining current issues in special needs provision
Catalogue update - new prices and availability on Touch Monitors
IT Fanzine - leave your comments in our guestbook
Who else is looking? - daunting data from a busy educational web site, plus a useful glossary of internet definitions
Free Resources and Updates - free clipart from some of our award winning software

Events

Forthcoming Events and Courses (UK)

Feature articles and special interest

International Special Education Congress 2000
NEW DfEE SEN Action Programme

Non-tables front page

©Inclusive Technology Ltd
15/4/99

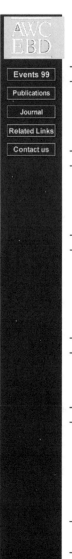

The Association of Workers for Children with Emotional and Behavioural Difficulties
A MULTI-PROFESSIONAL ASSOCIATION

What is AWCEBD about?

- **AWCEBD** exists to promote excellence in services for children and young people who have emotional and behavioural difficulties and to support those who work with them.
- **AWCEBD** has been active for over forty years. In 1992 it changed to its present name from the Association of Workers for Maladjusted Children.
- **AWCEBD** is concerned with children and young people of all ages in whatever setting their special need is found.

- **AWCEBD** is truly multi-professional, fostering the mutual understanding amongst the different professional groups that is essential to effective work. It supports workers in schools, mainstream or special, day or residential, Maintained, Non Maintained or Independent; in Social Service units, field or residential; in voluntary societies; in Health settings.

AWCEBD offers its members :

- **Information** to keep up-to-date with all the current changes in legislation and practice.

- **Support** of a quality that can only come from firsthand experience of this demanding work.

- **Help with professional development** at national, regional and group level.

- **A voice** to speak to central government, other public bodies and the media on behalf of children and young people with emotional and behavioural difficulties and of those who work with them. Our Scottish division offers the same service in relation to the statutory agencies in Scotland.

What AWCEBD provides

- **Journal** : our respected journal, "Emotional and Behavioural Difficulties", written for and mostly by practitioners on issues central to our work, is published three times a year.
- **Newsletter** : keeps members up to date on new legislation in our field. It circulates our responses to government consultation papers. It alerts members to relevant official reports.
- **Other publications** : we publish monographs and handbooks specific to work in our field.

- **Professional development** : our annual residential study course is celebrated for its professional excellence and for being friendly, supportive and sociable. It has lively format with prestigious lectures, working groups and special interest groups. it encourages participants to call together ad-hoc groups to share ideas on whatever concerns them. We have the annual David wills lecture, given by an eminent figure in our field. We have regional committees. We are developing training resources and can advise on in-service training.
- **Research** : We initiate and cooperate with research projects in all areas which relate to children with emotional and behavioural difficulties.

Who makes AWCEBD policy?

- **AWCEBD** is run by its members. A small Executive carries out the policies formed in National Council meetings held quarterly and attended by representatives of the regions. Officers are elected by the whole membership and all give their services voluntarily.

  Regions have considerable freedom to organise themselves as they wish. Many of them have open committees and welcome new members who want to contribute to the work.
  Members can get together to form new branches.

Why a separate special needs group?

- **AWCEBD** believes that the needs of children and adolescents with emotional and behavioural difficulties are not well understood either by society at large or by the public bodies who should provide resources. In our troubled society children and young people with emotional and behavioural difficulties form the largest and fastest growing special needs group. Resources to help them are inadequate and many of them are now at serious risk. Without the special help they need if they are to have the hope of a reasonable future.
- **AWCEBD** support parents who, unlike parents in other special needs groups, feel that they evoke very little public sympathy and do not form pressure groups. Nor do they assert their child's legal right to adequate help. If we who know at first hand the needs of these children and their families do not speak with a united and powerful voice we shall see wrong solutions enforced. Vital resources will be lost. So we need the strength that comes from our shared belief in a vital cause.
- **AWCEBD** is not isolationist. Our regions collaborate with other special needs organizations in holding events, in coordinating activities. We have been major partners in the two International Special Education Congresses held in the UK. We are founder members of Young Minds, the National Association for Child and Family Mental Health.
- **AWCEBD** membership is open to all those concerned with the education, care or treatment of children and young people with emotional and behavioural difficulties.

AWCEBD Publications   AWCEBD Events   AWCEBD Journal

Ring, Fax or Write to:
Allan Rimmer, Administrative Officer
Charlton Court, East Sutton, Maidstone ME17 3DQ
Tel: 01622 843104 Fax: 01622 844220

00789

APPENDIX 5

Individual education plans

This appendix contains examples of fictitious Individual Education Plans (IEPs) to illustrate plans at different stages throughout the Code of Practice. It also contains an example of commercially available material.

We recognise that many Early Years Partnerships and Local Education Authorities have also produced advice notes and examples of IEPs, and we encourage readers to look at local documentation to promote continuity of practice.

Example 1

Background information

Nathan is 4 and a half years old. He was born 9 weeks prematurely and experienced breathing difficulties at birth which restricted the oxygen flow to his brain. This has resulted in a general developmental delay. He started school with his peers at 4 years old and as his needs were assessed through the statementing process. His first Individual Education Plan is set out below.

NAME: Nathan   *DATE OF BIRTH*: 9.3.95   *DATE OF PLAN*: 7.9.99
NATURE OF CONCERN: General Developmental Delay

Overview of curriculum plan for half term
Curriculum designed to be working towards the Desirable Learning Outcomes. Theme to be built around 'Denny's Dream', designed to include imaginative work on what it would be like to be part of a different world. Language and literacy to be encouraged in all areas – including describing feelings of what it feels like to be different. Children to be encouraged to act out this story and improvise stories for themselves. Specific vocabulary to be highlighted and understanding confirmed by encouraging the children to use those words in different contexts. Familiar objects photographed from unfamiliar angles to be used to encourage questioning of what the children see. Creative pictures to be produced to illustrate the story and each child to produce a collage of themselves as part of the illustration. Maths to be

highlighted in counting body features, windows, doors etc. Perception of scale, how big are you? What is 'big'? Information and illustrations of various different environments to be collected and discussed. Children to make their own Denny from a choice of mediums – cloth, felt, different painting and drawing mediums, paper mache, plaster, sand.

Action – identify specific programme, activities, resources, staffing, frequency of provision, specialist help, involvement of parents, medical assistance	Evaluation – Records and reports	Initial targets – curriculum area and time scale	Review – identify date and who will be involved
One-to-one time of 1 hour to be spent with Nathan three mornings per week as follows: Monday Language and literacy Wednesday Help and support during physical activity Friday Specific help with numeracy	Parents to receive diary detailing specific activities Nathan has tried and suggesting support activities to do at home.	Nathan to learn six key words and show understanding and use in different contexts. Nathan to be encouraged to count from one to five both forwards and backwards by rote learning. Continued encouragement to use pencils/pens – at present grip results in variable control. Nathan to be encouraged to remove own shoes and socks during changing time and attempt shirt buttons. Nathan to be encouraged to play interactive games with other children during afternoon activity choice time – at present he is still keen to play solitarily. Nathan to be encouraged to use scissors. Various materials including playdough to be available to encourage satisfaction at using scissors. Nathan is reluctant to use scissors as he thinks he is bad	Informal discussions between classroom assistant and parents to take place fortnightly as agreed. Also, use of the diary. More in depth discussion including teacher at end of half term to review targets and achievement. Input from all adults and Nathan.

(cont'd)

Action – identify specific programme, activities, resources, staffing, frequency of provision, specialist help, involvement of parents, medical assistance	Evaluation – Records and reports	Initial targets – curriculum area and time scale	Review – identify date and who will be involved
		at it. Nathan to be encouraged to work with another child to feed the birds. This will involve regular trips to the nature area near the classroom. Sightings of birds are recorded on a chart with pre-prepared stickers. Both children are encouraged to tell the rest of the class what food they have been providing.	

Example 2

Code of practice record

Stage 1 – note of concern
Stage 2 – prepare learning strategies and targets
Stage 3 – involve outside specialists
Stage 4 – formal assessment with LEA
Stage 5 – formal statement of SEN
Name of child: Brian   *Age*: 3.6 years
Address:
Name person responsible for coordination of information:

Main area of concern
Attention control and aspects of behaviour which result in attention seeking. Lack of

conformity within a group situation. Behaviour that is inhibiting learning within the group. Immediate action: tasks broken down into smaller steps, reduction in group size, increased praise. This has lessened the negative behaviour exhibited by Brian. Parents informed of situation and aware of the need to observe and monitor his development and if appropriate carry out intervention strategies with regard to behaviour and learning.

Staff informed and consulted – yes

Parents informed – yes

A detailed observation of progress within the group followed initial discussion with parent. This was carried out in conjunction with staff and the coordinator. The report formed the basis of an individual educational plan which was presented at a staff meeting on 21.05.00. The agreed plan is shown below and parents will be consulted prior to implementation.

Staff members felt that Brian's behaviour had improved following reduction in group size and more attention to praise. It was felt that observation and monitoring should continue with regard to his behaviour and attention control within the group. Mrs Staff will record ongoing day-to-day response to learning (diary note form).

Strategies to be used by all staff and those who have contact with Christopher:

- Use all opportunities for praise, especially when behaviour is *positive*.
- Brian tends to break eye contact especially when he realises he has produced unacceptable behaviour and if an adult reacts with tone of voice or verbal disdain. He needs to strengthen his communication skills using eye contact and positive attention control as a medium to assist his behaviour. Try and make eye contact and use appropriate facial expression to reward positive behaviour.
- Use outside practical play as a focus for language and learning and to monitor behaviour in relation to cooperation with others.
- Cognitive development will be monitored by staff as part of day-to-day learning activities. In particular, counting games, symbol tracing using a variety of media, sorting and recognition of colours.
- Brian shows a preference towards left hand use. When handing him materials offer these in a way to allow him to make a choice of hand preference. Monitor response.
- Continue with small group work. Praise any attempt to conform to the will of the group. Monitor his response to changes in routines, especially at lunch time. Review in July.
- Offer praise and make sure we all use the same rules and offer a

consistent approach to managing his behaviour. In particular, when he self-corrects his behaviour and resolves any potential conflicts with another child.

- Speak with parents and use this report as a framework for considering consistency of approach at home.
- Introduce ongoing observation of Brian.
- Monitor progress. This will include recognising and recording positive behaviour as well as negative responses to learning.
- Monitor with one-to-one work.
- Ongoing staff records and verbal comments to be collated.
- Consultation with parents.
- Monitor at staff meeting July 2000.

Example 3

IEPI – Sally J.

In accordance with the requirements of the Statement of Special Educational Needs served on Sally J. (August 9th 1999) there follows her individual Educational Plan. This was devised by Joan Smith (Senior Nursery Assistant) and Ann Jones (Deputy Nursery Assistant).

Name: Sally J.
Address:
Professional contacts/other agencies:
Named person:
DOB:

Learning objectives (six months)

To ensure that language acquisition continues to progress
To ensure that Sally mixes with her peer group and is included in as many activities as possible
To promote concentration and respond to adult encouragement
To organise staff so that she has the appropriate attention to promote her learning
To encourage physical development
To develop self-help skills.

Strategies

Strategies to meet these objectives, on the basis of four (morning) sessions attendance per week. Progress to be reviewed each term.

Many strategies are used to support children as they attend the nursery. These include warmth, security, a recognition of individual skills and building positive relationships between children and staff. Sally will be encouraged to participate in a variety of activities suitable for developing appropriate skills of communication and learning through first hand experience. In order to monitor her progress special emphasis will be given to the following:

- Praise all attempts to use expressive language with an encouraging smile and to respond immediately. This to be done through 'doll play' introducing language such as cup, bottle etc.
- To play alongside one other child when introducing doll play. This will create opportunities to take turns. This will encourage Sally to relate to children in her group. Also introduce particular games with the intention of encouraging Sally to be aware of the children in her group.
- To introduce singing rhymes to encourage Sally to interact with the children in her group.
- To encourage Sally to sustain her concentration on an activity she finds motivating and enjoyable, for at least 5 minutes.
- To aid her cognitive development through sorting, beginning with two categories and increasing the number as appropriate.
- To develop Sally's gross motor skills with an emphasis on ball play – kicking, throwing, rolling and catching. Reward to be given by verbal praise and encouraging smiles. Some of these activities to be also carried out in pairs to encourage turn taking and social interaction. Fine motor skills to be developed through peg-sorting, use of painting and felt pens, crayons and pencils.
- To encourage (with adult help) the use of a cup.

Methods of recording

Direct observation by staff to record Sally's response to specific strategies. The use of criteria referenced language and communication recording sheets.

Parent and carers will be consulted and work in tandem with nursery staff to support educational strategies and record progress.

The Statement of Special Educational Needs recommends that advice is sought from speech therapist, physiotherapist and occupational therapist. This plan will be sent to each with a request for comment and advice. Copies of this IEP will be sent to Educational Psychologist and a date for visit to monitor progress as recommended on the Statement.

INDEX